THE GIFTS OF CAREGIVING

ALSO BY CONNIE GOLDMAN

Tending the Earth, Mending the Spirit:
The Healing Gifts of Gardening (with Richard Mahler)

The Ageless Spirit: Reflections on Living Life to the Fullest in
Midlife and the Years Beyond

Late Life Love: Romance and New Relationships in Later Years

Secrets of Becoming a Late Bloomer: Staying Creative, Aware,
and Involved in Midlife and Beyond (with Richard Mahler)

Who Am I . . . Now That I'm Not Who I Was:
Conversations with Women in Midlife and Beyond

Wisdom from Those in Care:
Conversations, Insights, and Inspiration

THE GIFTS OF CARE GIVING

STORIES OF HARDSHIP, HOPE, AND HEALING

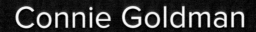

Connie Goldman

THE PARTNERS IN CAREGIVING PROJECT

CSA

Society of
Certified Senior Advisors·

THE SOCIETY OF CERTIFIED SENIOR ADVISORS

The Society of Certified Senior Advisors (SCSA) is the leading certifying organization for multidisciplinary professionals who have prepared themselves to work more effectively with older adults through education, training, continuing education and a professional code of eithcs.

Professionals who hold the competency-based CSA® designation have distinguished themselves by demonstrating knowledge and understanding of the multiple processes of aging that affect the biological, behavioral, social, and economic aspects of the life course. The CSA® certification is accredited by both the National Commission for Certifying Agencies (NCCA) and the American National Standards Institute (ANSI) meeting the highest standards of quality assurance available in personnel certification.

SCSA promotes knowledge exchange in the field of aging through traditional and new media channels including its award winning *Working With Older Adults* curriculum, the *CSA Journal,* educational webinars, conferences, workshops, newsletters, social media and local leadership groups.

Library of Congress Control Number: 2018931873
Second Printing 2018
ISBN: 978-0-9762451-1-7
Design: Stylus Creative
Printing: CEC Document Services Press

To all who are now or have been family caregivers. There is something in each of your stories that nourishes the strength and dedication needed to serve a loved one.

CONTENTS

FOREWORD

ISAK DINESEN, THE DANISH AUTHOR, ONCE SAID THAT ALL THE sorrows of life are bearable if only we can convert them into stories. This book is a collection of stories from caregivers, and the collection helps us to see how hardship can be converted into hope. But the magical power of this conversion remains hidden from us, a mystery we have not yet begun to unravel.

Paradoxically, this magic is hidden in plain sight, because the stories themselves are so clear and powerful that they speak immediately to the heart. We read the stories and are moved to tears. We recognize simple goodness, we are inspired by acts of kindness, and we come away even envying the storytellers, these remarkable people who cope with adversity in ways that leave us wondering, "Could I measure up to this challenge?"

What is hidden from us—the conversion of hardship into hope—is a mysterious element in the heart, an element that permits one caregiving relationship to be a kind of alchemy, transforming a base metal into gold, while another, faced with a similar challenge, causes bitterness and exhaustion. What accounts for this difference? What power in our own hearts could permit us to respond in such different ways to the imperative duties and impossible demands of a caregiving relationship?

The inspirational stories you will read in this book are other people's stories, and each one is unique. They cover a territory as wide as a caregiving relationship: from birth defects to Alzheimer's disease to an accident resulting in disability; from spousal obligation to volunteer caregiving to a child caring for a parent; from anguish to triumph to healed relationships.

The word *inspirational* may conjure up images of romantic glory—of someone like Mother Teresa rising from the slums of Calcutta to receive the Nobel Peace Prize—when we know too well that much of a caregiving relationship is drudgery, loneliness, and boredom. Above all, it is largely invisible. Caregivers are seldom celebrated in the public arena, and the person in care is simply now dependent. How does one cope with this invisibility? Those receiving care often have a limited voice regarding their choices. One doesn't need to become a world-renowned hero or hopeless victim, but each person must find his or her own path, own magical element, the alchemy that helps one escape resentment and frustration and find the gold in one's own heart.

Each of us, if we live long enough, can reasonably expect to encounter a caregiving relationship. Caregiving is our universal destiny. Very few people will reach advanced old age without being afflicted by chronic illness. All of us, as family or friends, will be touched by at least one person whose affliction falls into the category of hardship. We don't like to think about this fact, and so our current cultural infatuation with "successful aging" and "vital aging" insists that we keep these demons at bay.

Perhaps our cultural messages are wrong. Perhaps there are important lessons to be learned from a caregiving relationship, lessons about vulnerability, about our shared dependence on the kindness of strangers, about giving up illusions of control and autonomy. Both the one who is cared for and the one who gives the care face a challenge. Will we measure up? When our time comes, how will we respond to the challenge at hand?

If we think of life as a journey, then the condition of dependency can at any time interrupt our forward movement on this journey. A sudden stroke or a car crash, and life changes in an instant. We can't help but think, "It could have been me." Instead of a far-off destination, the journey suddenly becomes right here, in this bed, in this room, at this time. The journey of life, the forward movement, was perhaps always an illusion. When illusions fall away, we look for a new kind of hope. And the storytellers can provide us with that hope.

Journalists, like Connie Goldman, are constantly reminded to get the story straight. In turn, they remind us to get our stories straight: not to lie, not to deceive ourselves. The old-fashioned virtue of truth telling is the highest calling of the journalist, who is first and last a storyteller. What this collection of stories helps us do is get straight about the story of our own lives by reading the inspiring stories of those who have gone before us on the journey. For the transforming power of these stories we can only be grateful.

Harry R. Moody, PhD
Faculty Fellow, Fielding Graduate University

PREFACE

THIS BOOK WAS ORIGINALLY PUBLISHED IN 2002. IN EARLY 1999 I produced a one-hour radio program, *Hardship into Hope: The Rewards of Caregiving*, that was broadcast on National Public Radio. It consisted of a series of interviews with family caregivers—some well known and some not so well known but all with inspiring stories to share.

After *Hardship into Hope* aired, I was overwhelmed with letters, e-mails, and phone calls from people across the nation requesting printed transcripts and audiocassette recordings of the program. Listeners were inspired by the thoughtful words of Dana Reeve, wife and caregiver to actor Christopher Reeve, who had suffered paralyzing spinal injuries in 1995. They were moved by the insights of Ram Dass, the well-known spiritual leader whose stroke changed his role from caregiver to care recipient. They resonated with former first lady Rosalynn Carter's observation that nearly all of us will need a caregiver or need to become a caregiver sometime in our life. And they were grateful to hear positive stories of caregiving—stories of family intimacy, personal fulfillment, and spiritual growth.

Many listeners urged me to write a book based on the radio program. With their encouragement, I began to conduct additional interviews that put into words the special gifts of caregiving. The result is the book you hold in your hands, *The Gifts of Caregiving: Stories of Hardship, Hope, and Healing*.

When we read a book, we "hear" the words in our own voice, in our own head. My wish for you is that each story will bring you information and inspiration—that you or someone you know will be supported in transforming the hardship of caregiving into hope and healing.

ACKNOWLEDGMENTS

SERVING AS A FAMILY CAREGIVER REQUIRES A FULL-TIME MENTAL and emotional commitment. I give my thanks and appreciation to all who have shared their personal story with me and have given permission to appear in this book.

I'm also grateful for the help I personally received from the staff of my original publisher, Fairview Press. They contacted me in early 2000 and told me they had heard my public radio program sharing stories told by family caregivers. At that time the phrase *family caregiver* wasn't part of America's vocabulary. Of course, millions of people were providing such care, but it was considered a private matter. I'm grateful that Fairview Press recognized the significance of the topic before people began talking about it openly.

I offer a belated thank-you to former first lady Rosalyn Carter, author of the 1994 book *Helping Yourself Help Others: A Book for Caregivers*. That book begins:

> There are only four kinds of people in this world. Those who have been caregivers. Those who currently are caregivers. Those who will be caregivers. Those who will need caregivers. That pretty much covers all of us.

Her words gave birth to my efforts to collect and share the stories of family caregivers.

I hope you will find in these stories both hope and healing. As many of you have so often heard me say, "Facts illustrate, but stories illuminate."

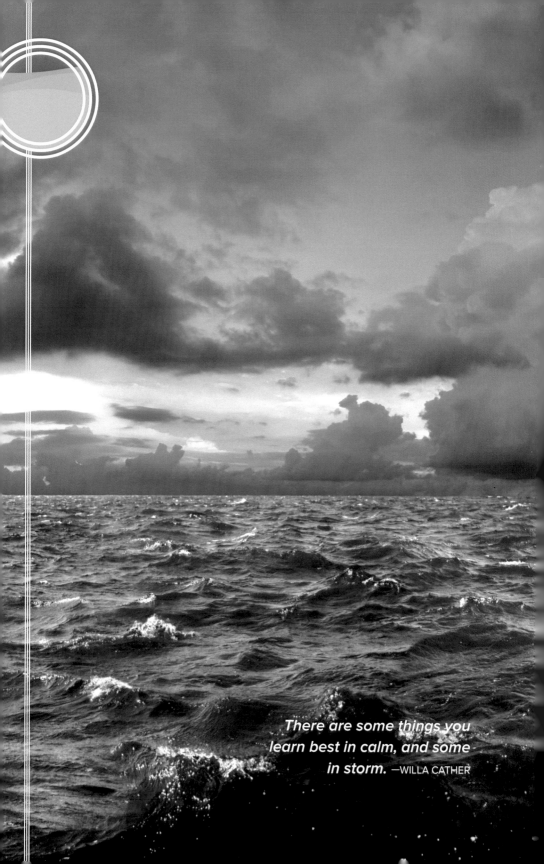

There are some things you learn best in calm, and some in storm. —WILLA CATHER

INTRODUCTION

MANY YEARS AGO I READ TEN WORDS THAT SHAPED THE direction of my career as a public radio producer, writer, and speaker. The poet Muriel Rukeyser wrote, "The world isn't made of atoms, it's made of stories." I had always been enchanted and entertained by a story. Thinking about the stories I had heard in my childhood and young adult years, I realized that in listening to these tales, I had discovered things about myself, my feelings, and my values. We have an opportunity to learn about ourselves from hearing the stories of others. Listening to people tell their stories and reading them, we laugh, we cry, we empathize. A story in a magazine or a newspaper deeply touches us. By sharing a personal and poignant tale, someone totally unrelated to our own situation may offer us an unexpected source of comfort and inspiration. We can gain insight and wisdom from someone we don't know and may never meet. Such is the power of a story, and that is why I'm sharing caregivers' stories with you in this book.

The personal narratives you'll read came from my meetings with a variety of family caregivers in various parts of the country. I talked with many middle-aged children dealing with aging, often critically ill parents. Some of my conversations were with spouses or companions whose mates were deteriorating physically and mentally. I collected stories that parents told about one or more of their children who required special care, and in some cases, would continue to require care over their entire lifetime. I recorded the experiences of people who had been caregivers for partners with AIDS; talked with family members who took care of cousins, aunts, or uncles; met with those who had assumed responsibility for the care of a friend; and spoke with several people who had taken over the care of a family member who lived a great distance away.

I traveled to New Jersey to hear the story of a woman who gave up her business and home and moved across the country to care for her frail and ailing mother. I went to Upstate New York to talk with a couple caring for two daughters who have been blind and physically limited since birth. I met a man in Maryland who lovingly cared for his wife as cancer drained her vitality. In Minneapolis I spoke with a woman who willingly assumed the role of family caregiver, first to care for her mother, then both her aunt and her uncle, because, as she explained, "I knew that if my mother were still alive, she'd be doing this for others in the family. I felt it was my responsibility to take over." A friend of mine in Maryland described in some detail what she called "a miracle of healing" between herself and her dying mother. A lifetime of abrasive and argumentative contact had evolved into unselfish caring, mutual respect, and deep love. I don't underestimate the healing power of reading such stories.

When my mother became ill and partially dependent, the word *caregiver* didn't exist. As nearly as I can determine, it wasn't in the dictionary until 1997. I didn't think of myself as a caregiver. I was simply a daughter who, when her mother required help, figured out how to provide the care that was needed. In my particular situation, my daughter and I became a caregiving team. I lived and worked almost two thousand miles away. I made the major decisions, provided suggestions from a distance, and flew back to my hometown nearly every Friday to relieve my daughter until I had to leave on Monday.

I remember wishing I knew someone else who was a caregiver, so I could talk about my involvement with him or her. In my circle of friends, I was the first middle-aged daughter to take care of an aging parent. My friends wanted to help, but my particular situation was outside the realm of their experience. I constantly juggled fear, frustration, irritation, indecision, and guilt that I wasn't doing enough for my mother and that I shouldn't be living on the other side of the country during her time of need.

At the end of her life, the most difficult thing for me was the sadness I felt not only because of the loss but also because some of the misunderstandings and unresolved issues between my mother and me were never openly discussed or repaired. Since then, people have told me many stories of difficult mother-daughter relationships that healed through a new closeness that arose in the caregiving relationship. I've also read several such accounts and continue to talk with people who have their own caregiver stories to tell. I believe all our stories can offer the gift of healing, forgiveness, compassion, and acceptance. We can learn from and grow through empathy for and understanding of others' experiences.

Among the many things I've learned from other caregivers' stories is that family caregivers often feel burdened, overwhelmed, and stressed. There's a good chance that a person who has taken on the responsibility of caring for another will experience feelings of depression, helplessness, and isolation. Yet we are far from alone. Dana Reeve, wife of the late actor Christopher Reeve, who suffered paralyzing spinal cord injuries, told me, "One of the things that I've realized is that I'm part of a group called 'caregivers,' and there are millions of us. It's often something that we take on willingly because we love the person and because we feel it's our duty, and yet we don't see it as a job, necessarily, and it really is. Not that we wouldn't do it anyway."

An estimated twenty-five million adults have added a volunteer caregiving commitment to an already full life. I've been told that only 13 percent of those requiring care are living in facilities that provide professional services. The other 87 percent live in their home or in the home of a relative. Their care has been taken on by family members or friends for whom caregiving isn't a paying job or chosen career. An estimated twenty-five million adults have added a volunteer caregiving commitment to an already full life.

We most often become caregivers through unforeseen circumstances. A father suddenly falls ill, a mother becomes increasingly forgetful, a spouse is diagnosed with a terminal illness, a grandmother is too frail to care for herself, an elderly friend is without family or resources, a child is born with severe physical or mental limitations. With little or no warning, we become caregivers.

We take on the role of caregiver because the alternatives aren't acceptable to our families or ourselves. Often, we don't know what we're getting into, but we make the leap anyway and hope for the best. Our day often includes dealing with frustration, stress, irritation, exhaustion, confusion, and guilt. Yet sadness and uncertainty are only part of the experience. Caregiving is also about knowing we've done our best and served someone we love.

Along with the awareness that a cure might not be possible and an acceptance of what can't be controlled or changed, many of us learn something deeply meaningful and profoundly spiritual about ourselves. Through the caregiving experience we can expand our vision, reach new depths of compassion and gratitude, and reassess our priorities. A daughter, herself in her sixties, reflected on the time when she sat with her dying, semiconscious mother. "Hard as it all had been taking charge of her personal care, seeing my own living patterns changed in almost every conceivable way, struggling with the guilt of never doing enough, still in some way I can't really explain . . . there's been some immeasurable value for me in just being there for her. Through this experience of caregiving, I think I've really grown and learned a lot about myself."

Many people I spoke with shared similar thoughts about a deepening personal awareness and growing sensitivity. Beth Witrogen McLeod, sitting in her sunny living room in Northern California, told me, "I think the ultimate learning in the giving of ourselves is that we find out who we are at heart. To give beyond any conceivable level than we ever thought we were capable of, or wanted to be capable of, or were willing to be capable of, is such a stretch of the heart. Still the opportunity to give to someone—that is the most healing, the most glorious connection that we can have as a human. You can't help but see the world differently. It changes you profoundly and permanently. It's a constant lesson to find out who we truly are." Beth wrote about her caregiving experience with her parents in her book *Caregiving as a Spiritual Journey.*

In several of my conversations, caregivers often told me how their priorities had changed—how they had gained new perspectives on what was meaningful in their lives and learned to slow down the pace of their days. Many spoke with a newfound sense of peace. I recall visiting with Gordon Dickman in Seattle. I was working on a different project at the time, and our appointment had nothing to do with caregiving. Yet, halfway through our conversation, Gordon shared his personal experiences about his father's death. "This is a story about holding an angel I didn't know was an angel," he began.

My father wasn't a man of words. He never said, "I love you," or "Son, you did a good job," or sat down and shared heart-to-heart talks with me. So, when he was in the last days of his life and comatose, and I was lying in bed with him holding him in my arms, I thought, "Why am I holding you in my arms like this? Why am I doing things for you that you never did for me?" And I began to reflect, during that long day until he died, on all the things he had done for me.

He'd driven miles when I was a child to take me to movies that I wanted to see. When I first started dating and couldn't drive a car, he'd driven into town, picked up the girl, taken us to the movies, gone somewhere and waited, come back and picked us up, and taken her home. And he never complained, never said no.

He's the one who drove me to college, set my trunk out at the corner, and drove off and waited at the end of the block until I went inside. I realized that he'd been there for me in my life all along.

And so, I could hold him and say, "I'm not giving you anything you didn't give to me, old man. I'm paying you back." And I held him until he died. I didn't let go, and I didn't let anyone else get in the way of that, either. I thought, "I'm not letting go of this angel until he's gone."

Is it trite to repeat that old adage "Every ending offers a new beginning"? I don't think so. Each story I've collected contains sound and sensible insights that offer hope and understanding and can nurture recovery and growth. Those I've spoken with often talked about the rewards of caregiving to describe their experiences. Some have actually called their personal growth a transformation. Others refer to what I've labeled the gifts of caregiving. Often these gifts aren't perceived or understood until after the immediate pressures and concerns of active caregiving are past. This learning has no particular time frame. Yet, sometime during our lifetime, whether we're the caregiver or the recipient of care, many of us will have an opportunity to explore the possibilities of transforming hardship into hope and to discover the incredible rewards and unexpected gifts of caregiving.

This book is about wives, husbands, life partners, mothers, fathers, daughters, sons, sisters, brothers, cousins, friends, neighbors—anyone who takes on the responsibility of providing care and comfort for someone who is ill, frail, or disabled. As you read the extraordinary stories of hardship, hope, and healing in this collection, I hope you will see that caregiving can be a gift in disguise, an experience that moves you toward a more meaningful connection with yourself and with others, and a chance to nurture your spirit and perhaps even to transform your life.

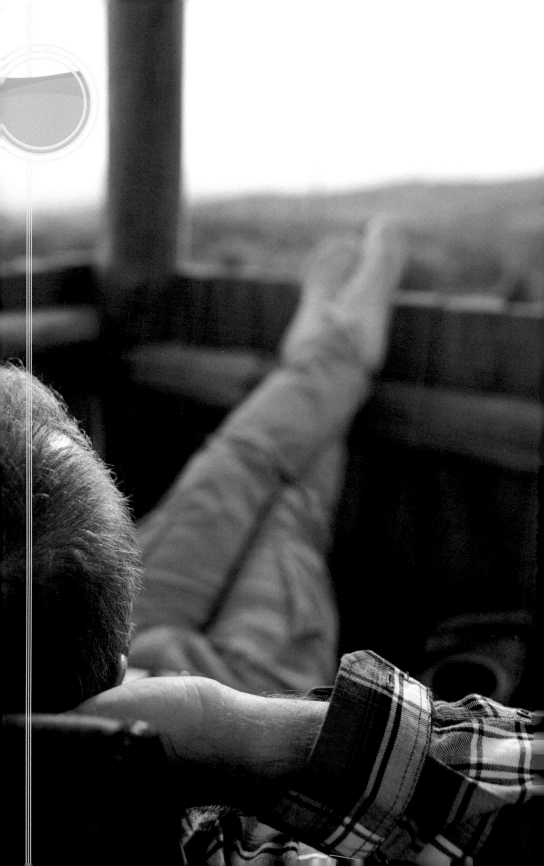

LEONARD

WHEN I'VE DONE SOMETHING FOR ME

LEONARD IS A PSYCHOTHERAPIST AND A PROLIFIC AUTHOR. ONE of his earliest books (still in print), *Here I Am: Using Jewish Spiritual Wisdom to Become More Present, Centered, and Available for Life,* reflects on what he and his wife learned about finding balance when caring for someone in their family. I read Leonard's book when it was published—when there were almost no books or other information specifically for family caregivers.

I later reread the slim volume—after I became a caregiver for my mother, who lived in a different city. It came to mind because I had been carrying tremendous guilt about having taken time for myself during my commitment as primary caregiver to my mother when she was fighting ovarian cancer. I felt overwhelmed as I tried to balance my caregiving situation and the demands of my employment.

Then one day I contacted Leonard, and we had a conversation about family caregiving. He began telling me his own story of serving as a family caregiver. His honest sharing is a reminder that both the one receiving the care and those giving the care need care. Yes, his psychiatric training was useful, but his basic advice to family caregivers grew out of his own personal experiences.

During those periods of my life when I was actively caregiving, I asked myself every day, "What do I need to replenish myself today so I don't feel completely like a victim?" I know you've probably heard others offer similar advice, but I'll repeat this thought now, because it's true and very important: caregiving requires taking care of yourself so you can take care of others. If I've done something for me during the day—whether it's walking or meditating for fifteen minutes, reading something that gives me pleasure, or just taking a hot shower or a relaxing bath—I feel less like a victim. When you're a hands-on caregiver, though, you give up some of your life. I think many caregivers give up too much, and then the task becomes totally consuming. I found that I was a better caregiver when I got a bit selfish. When I've nourished myself, I have more to give. I'd like to share some of my personal experience and learning that offered me and my wife some relief during the times we took on family caregiving responsibilities.

When I was ten years old, my mother found out that she had breast cancer. For the next four years she went through all kinds of surgery and experienced a dramatic series of emotional ups and downs. This was the most traumatic and powerful experience of my young life. I'm still reverberating from how intense it was for me. I've since gone through other caregiving challenges—my mother-in-law's leukemia, my brother-in-law's schizophrenia, and another close relative's Alzheimer's. Each time has been so intense that I have had to remind myself to slow down and breathe.

For some of us, guilt is always going to be there. We may think, "I shouldn't be doing this. I shouldn't be thinking of myself at a time like this. I should be giving care to the person whose care has been entrusted to me." This may sound strange, but I think it's the good people who feel guilt. People who are insensitive, narcissistic, and indifferent don't experience guilt. Feeling guilt is related to feeling compassion. I truly believe that the guilt a caregiver may feel is just part of being a compassionate, deeply feeling, sincerely caring, and loving person.

I often tell family caregivers, "You're allowed to know your limits." Sometimes the best way to honor your loved one is to know when you need to go to ask for help. Families don't talk about that much. Somehow the expectation is that the primary caregiver can handle whatever challenge comes along. I've found that rarely does anyone let you know it's okay to call in help—a nurse, a respite care person, a social worker, or another person who can do the things you're either not good at or that would be much more efficiently handled by another person. For example, there's an art to lifting a person to a sitting position. I can't do it. I'm not a weak person, but I can't do it without pulling my back out. I need to know my limitations. Taking on some tasks puts me at risk of becoming the patient! I'm not going to be a very good caregiver if I'm flat on my back.

I discovered a unique outlet for the pressure and tension that often come with being a caregiver. I had a friend who let me complain to him once a week. It was a huge relief. I urge others to do the same. I suggest finding a complaint partner—someone who will listen to you for ten minutes without interruption—and you return the service by doing the same. Anything and everything that's said during the ten minutes is okay.

My wife and I had another ritual. At the end of the day, we'd say to each other three things that went right that day. I remember one day when my mother-in-law was uncomfortable and the doctors were doing what doctors do, and we couldn't seem to connect constructively with any of them. The day was full of frustrations and worry. We sat down late in the evening and did what had become our ritual, searched for three things that went right that day. After what seemed a long silence, my wife said, "My mom smiled once today." I then offered, "The nurse who screwed up yesterday didn't today." We were having a hard time coming up with the third thing when my wife said, "We loaded the dishwasher and ran it, and now we have clean dishes." It makes a difference to experience three things going right, even if 150 things went wrong that day. You build momentum from that, find some peace of mind, and plant a seed of hope that tomorrow will be different.

It's interesting to observe how one person in a family often becomes the primary caregiver of a parent or other relative. Very often, a person who's either geographically or emotionally close to the person rushes in to help. The rest of the family empathizes and sympathizes, and the one person who takes on the caregiver challenge really needs the help and support. Too often that new caregiver, for whatever reason, doesn't ask others to help. The caregiver makes excuses for the others like, "This person is too busy, that one lives too far away, he has an important job, and she has those little children to take care of." When I was in that situation I discovered a way to honor the needs of other family members and also serve mine. I found out that everybody has something they're good at. I'm a good hand-holder. That's what I do best. My sister is good at paperwork. In some way all family members can participate without having the hands-on responsibility for the person needing care.

The need for caregiving often hits people very unexpectedly. And then we who take charge of the caregiving don't think to ask questions of those who have been down this road before. Too many people assume the job of the primary family caregiver and try to handle the situation and master everything alone. This attitude is just plain self-destructive, especially when there are organizations like Catholic Charities, Jewish Family Services, Lutheran Social Service, and so on. These people know so much. They're just waiting for people to call them so they can be of service.

For instance, when my mother-in-law was going through chemotherapy, we talked with a woman from a social service agency. She knew where to get shawls to help my mother-in-law feel like a beautiful woman when she didn't have any hair, where to get papaya drinks to calm her nausea, and where to get protein powder to help her get strong. They know how to deal with these things, and what to do when doctors have three different opinions, and how to handle financial confusion. There are people out there to help you and support you in these ways. But first, we have to break out of our shame or denial and share some of the problems (the so-called dirty laundry) with someone who's a stranger.

In spite of the problems and pressures, caregiving can offer great personal rewards. People don't always realize how much intimacy and closeness is possible. Just holding my mother's hand and feeling the connection between us was a very special thing. Some people may not have a good relationship with a parent, but when their parent becomes ill, the personality traits that caused conflict fade into the background, and they can often connect with the essence, warmth, neediness, and spirit of the parent for the first time. I think that often personality gets tossed aside by the illness, and you have a chance to connect with a person on a soulful or spiritual level, perhaps for the first time. I believe it can be one of the richest experiences in their life and in yours.

My mother-in-law, an anxious, agitated person her whole

life, was, in the last weeks of her life, open to being loved. And there was such warmth and connection. The day before she died, I just sat there and held her hand. This is something I never would have done before. She had never been open to that kind of thing, yet now she seemed to welcome it. If there's a situation like this in your life and if you have some way of connecting in a deeper way or a more conscious way, then I say grab it. It's something you'll remember for the rest of your life.

When you've been through this with someone, you really know how fragile we are. Then you start to appreciate how much in your body is working right, and you start to truly appreciate the miracle of human life. You start to realize what's really important. Caregiving gave me an opportunity to clarify what I wanted to devote my life to. I knew I didn't want to waste my life in a career that meant nothing deep and meaningful to me. I have had for several years now a personal life and work that gives me deep satisfaction and a sense of being of value to others. This is for me a high priority. Through my personal caregiving experiences I gained this perspective, and now it's part of my career.

Gifts can be found in the caregiving experience, even when the focus is on bathing someone, wiping a bottom, making a trip to the doctor, or doing one of a million different tasks of immediate priority. Even if you're enduring someone's violent outburst or experiencing their depression or unresponsiveness, there are ways to look for the grace in the experience of being a caregiver.

Caregiving is a great time to dig deep and find your Higher Power, your God, your faith. Many people use their spiritual energy to pray for a cure, but we shouldn't blame God if it doesn't happen. This spiritual energy could be put more constructively into a prayer that asks, "Please give me the strength to be open to possible connection with people who can help, and surround me with people who are positive, warm, and loving." I can also suggest one more prayer for a family caregiver: "Please help me to learn and grow from this experience."

Every family will probably at sometime deal with the challenges, stresses, and drastic changes that arise when a close relative requires care. So often the conversations focus on the care needed for the person who is ill or injured, now partially dependent or possibly requiring full-time care. The person taking on the primary responsibility of someone's care also needs to understand a principle that is often overlooked, that caregivers also need to care for themselves.

A family's focus is often primarily on the practical problems such as doctor consultations, costs of engaging extra help, the quickly changing needs of the person in care, and family decisions concerning who will assume what responsibilities and who will be available when the need is immediate.

Hopefully, more families in caregiving situations will come to understand the importance of care for the caregiver. Much of what Leonard shares of his personal experiences can be a source of encouragement for caregivers and can heal tensions and disputes in family conversations, and also enrich the primary caregiver's mental and physical health.

How does one justify taking this personal time? There was a time I was flying on an airplane, and the flight attendant gave the best caregiving advice I've ever heard. All of us have heard it, but none of us knew it was caregiving advice. She said, "Put on your own oxygen mask before helping the person next to you." Many of us would instinctively reach out to help the child, the person, the spouse, or whoever is sitting next to us before taking care of ourselves. The reality is that if you don't have adequate oxygen, you can't make good decisions, you get impatient, and you're just not in control. It's a reminder that we need to take care of ourselves first to do our best as caregivers.

1. What are your reactions and responses to Leonard's caregiver experiences and what he has learned from his personal caregiver experiences?

2. What stories can you share about caregivers who realize the need to care for themselves or who are not aware of the need for self-care and time out? What were the consequences of their choices? What stories can you share about family reactions and responses to the primary caregiver's needs?

3. What stories can you share about personal growth and meaningful learning that grew out of a family caregiving situation?

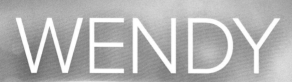

WENDY

GOING OUT ON SATURDAY NIGHTS

WENDY IS A THERAPIST AND COUNSELOR WHO OFTEN HELPS others deal with the stress and frustration they are experiencing as family caregivers. Many of her clients are members of that fast-growing population of middle-aged children with aging parents. I asked Wendy to share her personal experience and some of her thoughts and learning from counseling family caregivers. Our conversation began with some general thoughts about family caregiving.

A lot of people in their forties, fifties, and sixties who haven't yet been caregivers are terrified of it. They think, "Oh my God, what if my parents need me? What if my older sister or brother needs me?" They think caregiving is going to be a time of unmitigated horror and strain. They can't see the enrichments to the self that will accrue later. I like to tell people that there are many hidden benefits and not to run the other way when your chance comes. Go for it. It's being at a distance from illness, disability, or death that makes us so afraid. If you go up close to a thing and touch it, you learn the contours of it. It's not all one bleak world of horror. It's in service to others that we have an opportunity to learn and grow. Such possibilities are truly limitless.

One day, it was Wendy's turn to become a family caregiver. She and her husband decided to have his very ill mother move into their home.

It didn't take me long before I realized that my husband and I had stopped living our lives after my mother-in-law moved into our house. We stopped going to the movies on Saturday night. We didn't go out to dinner with each other, and our time in our own relationship had dwindled to almost nothing. I realized this wasn't going to work. So one day I said, "We have to start going out again on Saturday nights. We can't take away your mom's loneliness, and if we don't live while we take care of her, then we're waiting for her to die so we can live our lives again."

So, with a good deal of reluctance on my husband's part, we

began making plans for Saturday nights. The first few times were very, very stressful for us. It was hard to take our lives back, because it meant leaving her alone. It was painful. But after the third time we went out, she said, "Have a good time, kids," and gave us her blessing. When we'd come back from an evening out, it was good seeing her again and fun telling her what we had done and where we had gone. There was a sense that the oxygen had come back into the house.

Near the end of her life, my mother-in-law couldn't lie down at night. The cancer in her lungs made it too hard to breathe. Three nights in a row I sat with her all night, rubbing her back. I was getting more and more exhausted. Sometimes she'd fall asleep at four or five a.m., but this one night I was at the end of my rope. I'm a very patient person, but we were like little children, both so tired and aggravated. I said, "Well, if you won't lie down, then I'm going to lie down," and I just passed out. You've got to picture this. I was sound asleep diagonally across her hospital bed. The next thing I knew, I woke up and my mother-in-law was in my arms. Certainly in our waking state we would never cuddle. But I made sure I cuddled her really well as she slept. And in all my memories of caregiving, this was the most beautiful time. Even though she was asleep, I was very much awake, and I really got to hold her.

This experience had blessings I can hardly verbalize. I feel like I went to the edge of the wilderness and looked into it. It was a wake-up call. You learn after taking care of someone to bless literally every day that you're not homebound. I feel the privilege of enjoying a beautiful day, even being able to walk up my front steps. I have so many memories of helping my mother-in-law go down those very same steps. And in her delight in being out of the house she would see every flower, every little special garden arrangement, every pot, and every little statuette. My mother-in-law actually taught me how to see. She conveyed delight to me, and that gift of being able to really see in a new way and slow down has stayed with me.

We just don't make these observations in the hurly-burly of our busy lives. But the minute someone you love gets sick or suffers a devastating medical condition you say, "Whoa, what is life about? I'm just as fragile as this person lying in the bed. What am I doing? How am I living? What is the rest of the time that I have really for?" I think in our life today we almost need illness or something that slows the pace of our lives in order to become fully awake.

Taking on the responsibilities of a family caregiver often requires drastic changes in one's life. I know from others, and my own personal experience, that such changes are most often seen as negative. Some family caregivers modify work responsibilities, eliminate leisure activities, and in many situations provide living space in their home for the person in care. Such changes in one's regular pattern of living often involve losses. Indeed, the new caregiver responsibilities do absorb the time and energy previously given to other plans. Integrating these often dramatic changes is always a challenge.

The caregiver's awareness of the needs for self-care and for seeking a positive view of a situation can make a difference. Family caregivers have told me about a new unexpected relationship growing between them and the person in their care. Some have talked of the healing between them that they never anticipated. Others have revealed the discovery of a new depth of emotions. Some of us gain new perspectives by traveling around the world, while others discover profound insights in far more limited landscapes such as being a family caregiver. The person in care can often share thoughts and values that reveal more of who he or she is and, in the end, change the caregiver. Wendy's mother-in-law's slowing became the gift of her caregiving experience.

1. Have you seen a caregiver abandon intimate relationships or even everyday interactions with family members when assuming the caregiver role? If so, how have you or others dealt with these situations? What have you learned from them?

2. Caregivers are often forced to slow down their normal pace to accommodate the behavior of the person in care. Describe a situation where this has resulted in new awareness and deeper understanding for the caregiver.

3. What stories can you share that tell of interactions with the person in care that motivated changes in the thoughts and actions of the person providing care?

BILL AND JUDE

EVERYDAY LIFE TEACHES US

IT WAS WINTER, AND AN ENORMOUS AMOUNT OF SNOW HAD fallen in Upstate New York. Flights to Syracuse were being canceled regularly, so I decided to take the bus to visit with Bill and his wife, Jude. They live outside Sherburne, New York, with their five children. We talked about their work before we talked about the children. Several years before, Bill had started a movement called the Eden Alternative that has humanized hundreds of nursing homes throughout America. The changes include bringing plants, pets, and children into nursing homes and other living situations that previously lacked a homelike atmosphere.

On their property, adjacent to their home, they'd recently built a modest-sized, inviting retreat center where they host weekend seminars designed to explore ways of creating positive change in our society. According to Jude and Bill, "It's a place for intelligent and passionate discussion that plants seeds for change."

We sat at their kitchen table after dinner. Zachary, age twelve, and Virgil, age ten, were in the living room doing whatever young boys do to avoid paying attention to their homework. Caleb, the baby of the family, was already in bed for the night. Their daughter Haleigh, age six, was being fed strained baby food by a nurse; their other daughter, Hannah, age four, was lying in a special reclining stroller. The girls were exceptionally small, each weighing around thirty pounds. Both were born with Ohtahara syndrome, a malfunction of the nerve cells. Both are blind, suffer from seizures, are susceptible to respiratory infections, and require continuous nursing care.

You might expect their home to resemble a hospital or clinic, but you'd be mistaken. It has the warmth and charm of a country farmhouse. The room where Haleigh and Hannah sleep has an elegant bed with sides that come up to prevent the girls from falling out. An adjacent bathroom has been designed to accommodate a nurse who assists with all bathing and toilet functions. Their room is warm and cozy, decorated with dolls and other toys, although Hannah and Haleigh will never be able to play with them.

Everything visible looks like a typical young girl's room. Yet, this is not a "normal" situation. Jude served tea, and the three of us sat together looking through the large window as the snow fell outside. It was time for conversation. I listened while they talked about their heartaches and their joys. Jude began.

Both of our little girls have Ohtahara syndrome. This disease is so rare that there are only thirty known diagnosed cases in the world. It took about six weeks before we realized something was wrong. Then we were told there was no cure. They told us Haleigh would not live six months. The doctors told us the syndrome wasn't genetic and that we could have another child. And then Hannah was born, and within twenty-four hours she had a seizure and we were headed down the same path. The issue is with my eggs. We have two older boys who are my stepsons, so they're well. Sometimes I look at the girls and think it's all my fault. It hurts.

It's my personal struggle. We chose to have an egg donor for our last child.

When my first daughter, Haleigh, was born, I was devastated. When I found out she wasn't neurologically normal, I didn't know what that meant. Once I understood, I withdrew from the baby and didn't want to touch or hold her. I chose to disconnect because I was told she wouldn't live past six months. And then something changed, and I scooped her into my arms and knew I'd love her. I still feel horrible about this. What a difficult adjustment that was! The most important lesson for me was to mourn the child I didn't have. Before you can accept what you get, you need to mourn the loss of your expectations. When I'd see a child the same age, I'd cry. Yet eventually I let go of what I thought would be a normal life with a normal child.

The girls live with and are part of the family. We made the decision that we weren't going to run around to doctors looking for miracles, so we just brought each of them home when they were born. People say we are such special people to do this. We're not. You do what you have to do. Having the girls has made me realize that I'm a lot stronger than I ever thought I could be. If you had told me when I was in my twenties that I'd have two children like this and I could live with the situation, I would have thought you were crazy. But you handle it; you get up in the morning, and you just do it.

Neither of my girls can talk or see. They can hear music; they can smile and react. And they can show us when they are sad. That's the hardest thing for me, because they can't tell us why. That hurts. I wish they could talk. But we just try one thing and another, and eventually something works.

We didn't want our home to look like a hospital. We have the things we might need, like oxygen and other medical equipment. But we've made special beds that look nicer than hospital furniture and a special bathroom and shower. Sure, you can tell that both girls have special needs, but our home isn't set up like that.

We have round-the-clock nurses. Our nurses are exceptional; they're an extension of our home and like our family. They share both our joys and our sorrows. We really want our daughters to be with us and to be part of our family. They used to call children such as our girls "throw-away" babies. They'd go to an institution, without being given a name, without being given the care they needed, and they'd perish. One of our nurses said to me one day, "Your girls are alive because of the love you give them." I believe that's true. Our love, the love of our other children, and our nurses' love make all the difference in our world and theirs.

This is the kind of thing you've got to deal with directly. There's no way of hiding or covering it up. Our marriage was challenged, but we're strong now, and so solid. A friend of ours had a disabled child around the same time Haleigh was born. The baby died, and, sadly, the marriage was ruined. I really don't know our secret. But I do know that something like this can actually make a marriage and a family stronger.

Then Jude's husband, Bill, joined the conversation.

Our biggest fear is that we will run out of funding for nursing care. But we'll figure it out, because we'd never put the girls into an institution. We ensure that as a part of our family they have a life of peace and tenderness. There is joy to be found and love to be felt no matter what they can or can't do.

I spend a lot of time speaking to nurses and doctors about caregiving. Even if I don't specifically mention my girls, what

I say is informed by my experience at home. It has made me a better physician and teacher.

Our two older boys don't realize they're having a childhood experience unlike any other. Just last Saturday they had friends come over to play, and the boys just casually said to their friends, "That's Haleigh, and that's my sister Hannah," and then they zoomed on to the next thing they were doing. Once we went to a public playground, and my young son saw that the handicapped swing was far removed from all the others, and he asked why they would do such a thing. They're growing up without a sense of shame or remorse about the life they live. Our boys are more accepting of others' differences, and that's carried over to all kinds of people. That's a real gift of learning. I actually think they're growing up wiser souls.

Our daughters survive with the help of a lot of potent medications, but we deliver them in a context of love. A cruel truth of caregiving in America is that we have reduced the idea of caregiving to providing medication, therapy, and exercises. This is part of the story, and we can't deny the value of medications, but it's not the whole story.

Here's a little irony. Let's say you are taking care of someone, and you pour out your heart and soul and give your love and tenderness. Let's say they get better. One of the first things that happens is that the financing service, the insurance company or whomever, will kick the ladder out from under you. The system came back to us and said, "Look, your girls haven't had to be hospitalized for a time now. They're okay, right?" And we say, "That's because the financial help allows us to get good nursing. That's how we've kept them out of the hospital." Nevertheless, they remove the supports that have allowed things to get better and take away one of the key elements of success, making it much more difficult to continue the care. It's hard convincing anyone unless you've lived this. Yet, it's more than a personal problem; it's a political problem in American society.

At this point in our conversation, Bill had to leave for an appointment. Jude and I continued to talk.

We really want to see change in our society. I want people to start looking at and accepting people with disabilities and children who are different from other children and stop turning away. People will say how beautiful one of our "normal" children is and will just pass over our girls and look the other way.

Our work and our teaching is about understanding how important it is that a society provides for and organizes itself to meet the needs of the frail and disabled in the most humane way, so we have a better society for everybody. Our calling is to create a more engaging, forgiving, caring, and warmer culture. Caregiving for our girls has taught us a lot about this. You don't need to be a family caregiver to understand these needs, but we've learned a lot from our personal experiences.

Nobody comes into a caregiving or care-receiving situation on a voluntary basis. The truth is, we come to it kicking and screaming. All of us. What we have in our own home is a microcosm of how we'd like the world to work. Of course, many people don't have to think about these things right now, but it seems that everybody gets to some version of where we are sooner or later. Look around. It touches everybody. Family care issues are something everyone, everywhere, in some way will have to deal with.

Our home is the absolute center of our universe. Caregiving for Haleigh and Hannah has put the focus on our work here at home. A huge part of what allows us to do our work professionally is that we live it every day. Everyday life teaches us, and then we teach others from our hearts, from our experience; our girls come into our teaching always.

You asked us what we've learned from our personal caregiving experience. Well, we've certainly learned about the importance of living one day at a time. And our experience has shown us what a strong marriage we have. You learn little things every day, not always astronomical stuff, but the awareness of small things: the joy of going out for a walk, the pleasure of seeing how the trees look covered with snow.

And then there's the big stuff, the constant and unremitting reminder that you love your children just the way they are. There's joy to be found and love to be felt no matter what. We're thankful for everything we have. And maybe the girls are thankful too, in their way, for lives that are filled with peace, joy, and tenderness. They suffer some physical pain, and that's hard to watch. We struggle with this, because you always hear that God never gives you more than you can handle. But why us? Why them? It was hard to accept. But they are loved and they know that, and the rest falls into place.

There's a lot of love here, and that's the gift.

––––––––––––

The loving commitment of Jude and Bill to the lifetime care of their two totally dependent daughters certainly earns our empathy and sincere admiration. Their story is unusual and most likely different from the circumstances each of us is dealing with now or will face in the future. But no matter what challenges we face, all of us require time and the comfort and suggestions of others to accept our circumstances and form a workable plan for dealing with them. Painful and stressful as the situation may be, we need to believe that we can learn and grow as we work through possible solutions. I also believe we need others to help us when unexpected events occur. Family members, friends, neighbors, professional helpers, community organizations, religious communities, and other resources are available. Primary family caregivers need to reach out, recognizing they might be in their particular situation for the long haul.

1. Have you ever been in a situation where an accident, unexpected diagnosis, or other drastic change occurred in your family? If so, how was it managed?

2. What suggestions or guidance can you offer to keep emotions under control so sensible solutions can be arrived at? Do you think such situations require one person to take charge of the planning? If so, how can this be successfully accomplished?

3. Have you dealt with a situation where the attitude of an immediate family member was primarily negative? Have you been able to help the person modify his or her outlook? Has any change you've suggested changed the attitude or behavior of the person receiving care?

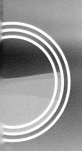

ELIZABETH

IN THIS THING TOGETHER

ALTHOUGH ELIZABETH AND HARRY BOTH HAD CAREERS AND were raising two young children, they took on the unique challenge of becoming caregivers not for a family member but for an elderly friend, Mr. Morris. While many people take on the responsibility of care for a relative, it's uncommon for a busy couple with young children to assume the full-time care of a friend. Mr. Morris was in his nineties, had outlived two wives, had no children, and was living alone in an apartment not far from Elizabeth and Harry. For many years, Mr. Morris had been close friends with the couple and had become like a grandfather to their children. He began having meals with the family quite frequently, and over the course of a year discussed the possibility of moving into an apartment adjoining their home that he would pay to construct. The addition was planned and built, and Mr. Morris moved into his new quarters and became a part of the family. Elizabeth tells of this unique experience of caregiving.

My husband and I wanted to give something back for all we had been given in our lives. We talked it over and decided to ask Mr. Morris if he would like to come and live with us. We really wanted him to be here, and we were ready to assume the responsibility of the care he needed. At that time, our longtime family friend was about ninety-one. He'd outlived everybody he knew; he had never had any children. When his late wife had had a stroke, he was her caregiver for three years. Now he needed someone to make life comfortable for him.

We built an addition onto our house—his own little apartment where he had his own kitchen and privacy. Mr. Morris stayed with us for six years. During the first few years he was quite independent. He did a little driving, and he usually would fix his own breakfast and lunch. He would join the family for dinner. For him to spend time with our young children, something he had rarely done, was a wonderful opportunity, a great thing for the children, who loved him dearly. It was just fine with them that Mr. Morris had all the time in the world, not like their parents, who were always in a hurry to get somewhere or get something done.

Gradually Mr. Morris became somewhat frail, and during the last year he was with us he was bedridden or in a wheelchair. We became full-time caregivers, as he then required a great deal of care. Fortunately, we have a large group of friends, and Mr. Morris knew many of them. An old friend of his was a nurse and lived only a few blocks away. Another was a physician who made house calls on Mr. Morris. Two or three men we know would take turns bathing him. So, we really didn't do this all by ourselves. We had the very meaningful support of a large group of friends who were also caring people. This provided respite for us. We had all the bases covered.

My time with Mr. Morris taught me a great deal. We talk of how important it is to live in the moment. Sometimes we say this blithely, not really understanding what it means. But when you're forced by your circumstances to slow down your life to the pace of someone who really does live in the moment, it changes your life. I would wake Mr. Morris up about 9:30 in the morning, and it would take me until about 11:30 to get him his breakfast, dress him, comb his hair, help him with his teeth, and situate him in his wheelchair so he could sit comfortably. But in those two hours, we would live each moment. I found it a humbling experience to discover I had to learn that.

At times I gave in to impatience and irritation, and I'm sure the tone in my voice wasn't gracious or kind. I'd hear myself saying something that was irritable and impatient, and that would snap me back into the reality of the situation. I knew this thing we were going through together could be horrible, a drudgery, or that together we could make it a deeply meaningful experience. Remembering that made it easy for me to treat Mr. Morris with kindness. He too would bring kindness and consideration into the morning. I'd be cranking up his bed, which was physically difficult, and he'd often say something like, "Oh, that's such hard work for you; I hope you don't hurt your back. Please be careful." In such caring exchanges, we made our interactions more than a morning of chores. The reality was that Mr. Morris and I were partners, we were in this caregiving thing together, and we learned from each other.

I discovered you can approach each moment in many ways. We all do so much in our lives that ultimately doesn't have much meaning. I think if you can focus on the present and truly know the value of doing something for someone that's good, something this person really needs right now, and you can do that good thing, everybody wins. I'm speaking about the essential quality of goodness, not excellence. I'm finding it difficult to explain this. I just know that service to others expands one's life and adds beauty. There's a man who lives on my street, a retired scientist, and every day I see him out walking and pushing the wheelchair of one of our neighbors. I see them walking and talking and enjoying one another. I feel I have a bond with this man. He understands.

As I look back on it now, those were the best years of my life. Caring for Mr. Morris was a blessing for us, an absolute gift. You know, people don't have that many opportunities to give back, and this was ours. Mr. Morris would not have had the comfort and dignity he deserved if he hadn't come to stay with us, but we were the winners in this situation. It's easy to be helpful when the need is clear. The way I try to live my life, I see service as a gift. I had the opportunity to step in and help, and that truly was a gift.

My conversations introduced me to unexpected connections growing between neighbors, club members, and others who establish relationships based on similar interests, hobbies, and newly formed book clubs but who may never have connected before aging became a factor. For Elizabeth and her family, Mr. Morris was first a friend and then evolved into a resident, a family member, and finally someone who required assistance and care. As they redefined their relationship, they found that caregiving can change both the pace and the understanding of such responsibilities. Assuming the responsibilities of a caregiver was an experience for Elizabeth that not only served Mr. Morris well but also gave her a new understanding of the time and commitment necessary to provide appropriate care. Her description of her caregiver day with Mr. Morris has become, with variations, the routine for several thousands of family caregivers in America today.

As I have so often said in speeches and in print, we need to consider ways to provide financial support for the many caregivers who give up jobs and earned income, and their independent life, when they devote their days to their caregiver commitment. I'm hopeful that in the near future state governments will consider legislation that would compensate families unable to give up the income from an outside job but also unwilling to leave a family member without the necessary care. This situation is no longer rare in the United States. The number of families having someone in need of home care is quickly mounting. Let's not only hope but also do what we can to educate and influence both local and national governments of this growing need, and offer suggestions for new services that could be provided for needy families. I believe it's a challenge that communities need to take on, and quickly.

1. **Who do you know who has given up a job to become a family caregiver? What has the caregiver compromised in order to take on this responsibility? Who has the caregiver approached for support and help? How have neighborhoods become part of a caregiving network?**

2. **Elizabeth needed two hours each morning to get Mr. Morris**

dressed, fed, and settled for the day. What stories can you share about what a caregiver commitment often entails?

3. Many who haven't had the experience or exposure to a caregiving commitment and responsibility have no understanding of the time and energy necessary to devote to such an obligation. How could you, along with fellow caregivers, take on the mission of teaching others, especially local governing groups and funding sources, about the time and energy necessary to fulfill such an obligation?

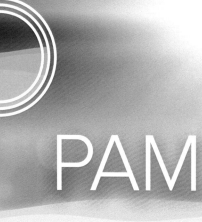

PAM

I ENTER HER WORLD

PAM HAS A FULL-TIME JOB MANAGING A LARGE COMMUNITY-based agency. Her public life in itself could be totally consuming, yet she deliberately makes adequate time for her private life, which includes a husband and children. Recently she has assumed the responsibility of caring for her eighty-eight-year-old mother who now resides in a nursing home not far from her office.

Recently Pam wrote an editorial for the local newspaper, "It's a Gift to Participate with Mom in Her Process of Aging." The first question I asked Pam when I had an opportunity to talk with her was why she wrote the piece. She replied, "I didn't know anything about dementia and how to deal with the changes in my mother's behavior. It's been such a profound and stunning experience for me that I needed to write about it. I believe what I learned can help others." I heard passion in her voice as she shared her insights.

My mother lived alone in her own home in another city and drove a car until about three years ago. When she began to show signs of confusion, she went to live with my sister. Now that I've taken on the responsibility of my mother's care, I often reflect on what it was like for my sister to manage her care for as long as she did. I can remember when we first noticed that my mom was acting strangely. She lost the ability to cook. She'd try to make her favorite dessert and ingredients would be missing or it would be burned. She'd try to make cookies that she'd made a hundred times before, and she couldn't do it.

Mother always had kept a meticulous checkbook, but when we went through her check register, we found she had completely lost control of paying bills and writing checks. This signaled to us that something was really wrong. We could see we were dealing with some kind of dementia. After one visit the doctor labeled it Alzheimer's.

One of my biggest revelations about Alzheimer's, or dementia of any kind, is that there's no point in attempting to adjust the perception of reality with someone who has dementia. I learned quickly that arguing or correcting my mother upset her, and me too. I wrote an editorial for our local newspaper and discussed this as my main point. I've found that acceptance is easier both for me and for her. I'll read you a paragraph from that editorial:

When my mother and I talk and her mind is clear, I rejoice in the give-and-take, the chance to tease her and even to get her to smile. When her mind is fuzzy, I appreciate the opportunity to just be there and listen, getting her to smile, and helping her to reenter the world and connect with me. When her mind is completely gone, I actually enjoy entering her fantasy world and I go with her where it takes me.

My mother likes to talk about having just seen her mother and my grandmother, who has been dead for several decades. Sometimes she tells me that she's walking down the hallway, she's going back to her hometown, she brought my mother a stuffed animal, and other things like that. As long as her delusions aren't frightening or harmful to her, I've learned to let go. I just play with it, and we have a fanciful conversation within her reality. What does it matter if it isn't my reality? It works for me to enter into hers. I feel best when I just go with it.

Yet sometimes she is very clear in her thinking and my mother is back with me. For a short while she has complete recall, and when that happens it's really fun. She never used to demonstrate affection, and now we often have tender moments when she'll let me hold her hand. Sometimes I'll have my arm around her and she'll put her head on my shoulder, and we have a sweet and close moment. She never would have done that when she was her old independent self. That just wasn't her mode when she was more in control of her behavior.

Mom isn't happy most of the time, but seeing familiar faces cheers her up. Our family has a lake cabin, and when we take her there and when family and friends show up, it makes her very happy. My sister got married this past summer at the lake, and we made a big deal about the wedding, partly for my mom, because it was a way to ask a lot of people to come see her and be with her. Frankly, from the day the wedding was announced, it was her entire focus.

I know too when I go to visit her, which is at least three times a week, it makes her happy. She has wonderful care in the place she's in now, far better than the first nursing home we had her in, but she doesn't seem to respond much to her surroundings. She's very much aware of her losses—the loss of her independence, her home, her car, and control over her money. Although she's aware of all these things, she can't really put together what has happened to her. She understands that everything has changed, but she doesn't have the ability to analyze it.

My husband and my two children (ages nineteen and twenty-three) have been wonderfully supportive of me, really giving me a place and space to process this. When I come home and tell my family about my visit with Grandma, they might be bored, but thankfully, they always let me talk. They've shared both my laughter and my tears. My tears come mostly from physical exhaustion. There was a time when my job was more difficult and demanding than it had ever been, and, between that and my mother, I got to a point where I cried for about a month. I just couldn't balance everything.

Another time of tears came when my mother was in a different nursing home. I was beside myself with grief and anger, and I couldn't control anything that was happening. Fortunately, that's not where my mom is now, but it's where she could be. Many caregivers feel helpless to get the care they want for their parent. I was very frustrated with Mother's lack of care, and my tears were about the whole institutional approach, the bureaucracy, and the fighting over medical systems, money, poor food, lousy care, and smelly hallways. My tears and exhaustion were more about the fights to get adequate care for Mom than the deterioration of her functioning.

We're in a culture that has not yet thought this through. Our society, which already has so many older people that need nursing home care, has just not planned for what it's going to take to care for the frail and elderly in the future. I know these problems can't be solved easily, but shouldn't there be a way to make humane care more widely available?

I'm conscious of wanting to model something for my kids. I hope my children will hang in there with me when I'm old and in need of care. Helping me with my responsibilities for my mother I know will make a difference in how they view things. Before this, my kids knew their grandma the way other kids know their grandmas. They visited her a couple of times a year, she baked them cookies, and they didn't particularly let her into their lives. They liked her fine because she was their grandma, but they didn't have a deep emotional attachment. So now they have a chance to really know her.

One Saturday night, for example, I was out with my husband, and my younger daughter was home with a friend. They were about to go out to a party when Grandma called. She was clearly distressed and needed somebody. My daughter went right over there with her friend. In some ways that seems like a little thing, but in this culture for a teenager to give up her Saturday night, when she was about to go party with friends, and respond first to her grandma's needs—well, that's something, I think. It was an incredible night, because instead of spending ten minutes with Grandma, my daughter stayed more than two hours. She ended up reading inspirational verse to her. The words probably meant very little to my daughter, but she figured out that this would be calming and meaningful to her grandmother. Even though it was only one experience, I think it was an important lesson for my daughter. When we discussed it that evening, I could see she got a lot from it. It was a lesson in compassion and understanding, a real gift.

I'm learning something about living, something about being a human being, that I might never have learned if this hadn't happened. My sister couldn't do it anymore, and we had run out of options. Moving Mom close to me wasn't well thought out. My mother just landed in my town and in my life. I didn't choose it, but I now consider it a miracle that it happened. I didn't understand or appreciate then what the caregiving experience could give to me. I truly feel grateful that the circumstances were such that I almost didn't have any choice but to take her. I don't want to romanticize this situation, but I've come to believe that becoming my mother's caregiver has been a real gift. I think about some of my friends whose mothers died without a prolonged physical or mental degeneration that required caregiving. On the one hand, they missed the really difficult process of decline, which is horrific; but on the other hand, they missed the opportunity for this very special relationship I have had.

As a caregiver, you really have to stay in the present. If you're distracted and aren't in the present, it's really an awful task. You can't think of what you have to do outside of being there. It doesn't matter what should have been or could have been, because it just is what it is. When I'm with my mom, I have to let go of the world, enter the nursing home, and just be there for her. None of the time orientation that runs our lives means anything to my mom. All she cares about is that I'm sitting there with her now. It's wonderful to realize that if you let yourself stop and just be there in the present for someone who really needs you, that's a lot for a human being to get in life. It's a tremendous gift, just to make someone really happy.

We don't often feel like we've made a difference in the world, but this is a very concrete way to make a big difference. Often when I'm busy with work and other things in my life, I make myself visit Mom. I don't really want to, because I've got a lot of deadlines for my job and I'm really hard-pressed for time. So sometimes I go to visit her with a bit of an edge, and then I spend a couple of hours with Mom, and I walk out and say to myself, "What was I obsessing about? This was a really nice thing for both my mom and me. It's given me something back that's really nice," and I leave the nursing home smiling.

Many friends, neighbors, and relatives have shared with me their experience of adjusting to a loved one who no longer shares their reality. Just as we correct a child when perception of some reality isn't accurate, it seems that often the immediate response to someone with some kind of dementia is to correct them as well. However, it's not the parent who needs correction; it's those who think they know what is going on. It's often a difficult behavior to learn because it demands some unlearning. The normal and immediate response to correct what seems like a verbal mistake must be accepted and passed over. A smiling acceptance and agreement opens the door to a comfortable visit and gradually a realistic acceptance of whatever form someone's dementia takes.

Certainly some other behaviors accompany memory changes and require various methods of limiting activity. Yet caregivers must control their desire to normalize the person with memory issues. I was glad that Pam also shared an honest view of her emotional exhaustion. Caregiver responsibilities along with the normal pressures and obligations of work and family can cause caregiver burnout. I've known of caregivers who wore themselves out both physically and emotionally. A few actually required hospitalization. Such a situation can complicate everything, so it is important that caregivers and their family be aware of the symptoms.

1. How have you or someone you know needed to adjust when a person in care presents behavioral changes, mood alterations, anger or demanding behaviors, or other such challenges? What have you learned from such situations?

2. How might you help family caregivers dealing with unexpected changes in their loved one's memory, mood, or behaviors?

3. When have you experienced the positive part of a seemingly totally negative situation?

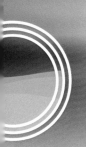

MARTHA

JUST TODAY IS ENOUGH

A MAILING FOR A DAYLONG SEMINAR SPONSORED BY THE LOS Angeles Caregivers Resource Center indicated the speakers would be family caregivers. Of course, that was of interest to me, so I registered for the event. The first speaker was Martha. The Los Angeles Caregivers Resource Center provides family caregivers with referrals, personal advice, and other types of assistance. When Martha left her husband, the agency helped her locate services for her paralyzed adult daughter, Janice, and provided counseling as Martha's personal situation and Janice's care needs changed. Martha told her story to an attentive audience, giving them hope and inspiration. I think her story, briefly retold here, will inspire you too.

I have three children. My son, Daniel, is twelve years old, my daughter Sara is fourteen, and my daughter Janice just turned thirty. In December of 1997, Janice was injured in a car accident. She suffered severe head trauma that left her nonverbal, noncommunicative, and nonambulatory. That was the beginning of a new way of life for us. I tried to make it all work—caring for the younger children, becoming a full-time caregiver for Janice, and holding up my end of the marriage. Janice's dependence had a great impact on a family that was already having difficulties. Eventually I separated from my husband, and I've now filed for divorce.

I have a huge family. Unfortunately, and incomprehensibly so to me, not one member of my family could bear to be with Janice after the accident. Some of them came once to the hospital, and even that was too much. It was easier for them to pretend that Janice and I didn't exist anymore. That was very painful for me. My mother did try to help, but she treated Janice like a two-year-old. My mother felt that's what you do. When Janice would do something out of her control, my mother would scold her, and then we'd all be upset. My mother didn't understand; it was causing too much stress. Finally she stopped coming. My husband's family kept telling me to put Janice in a home. They said that she'd gotten herself into the accident and we shouldn't spend our lives taking care of her. The tension in our house was terrible. When my husband came home, Janice and I went into her room and just stayed there. That was the beginning of my realization that things had to change.

Now my children and I are no longer living with my husband,

and I can function without worrying about his reactions. I'm free to spend the time I need to care for Janice. This isn't a small thing, handling all this alone. I'm an around-the-clock caregiver, and it's an adjustment every single day. We don't know what the day will bring. It's a very different life from other mothers and daughters. Janice has to communicate with her eyes. That we've learned together to communicate this way is the greatest joy. Janice doesn't have words to use, so I've found other ways of reaching out to understand what she's feeling. I've been putting energy into improving my communication with each of my other children, spending time with them, even if it's for short periods when I don't need to be with Janice. I share their lives in new ways. I've learned how to be a silent support for Janice and be there for my other children too. In a way, Janice has blessed us all with a new and different learning. Yes, the way we live now is a changed life. Janice and I have a partnership.

Being a caregiver has taught me to have small goals, a one-day-at-a-time philosophy. I've learned from Janice about patience, about reaching out of myself to others. For a long time I had only tears of sadness. Now, although I can't really explain it to you, they are tears of joy. I've made a decision. No matter what, my daughter is alive and every day is a celebration of life. I stop and realize what beauty there is in life and then look at the challenges we have and what it's going to take. I know I can find ways to help myself, to care for my other children, Sara and Daniel, too. You do have to be realistic. At some point, you are no longer hoping for full recovery, expecting a miracle. I think then you begin to set reasonable goals. Each day gives me strength and courage, and each day brings blessings. Joy is when I see Janice smile. It's simple things that are my hope and strength. Just today is enough for me.

This change in my life, becoming a caregiver for Janice, has brought me a gift of self-confidence, love, and appreciation, despite the obstacles that will continue to face me and my children. A professor of mine once told me that we have a choice—to open the windows of our mind and let the sun and the warmth and the love come in. The choice is about what we do with what we've got to deal with. I'm not letting anger, bitterness, sadness, or depression overwhelm me and overtake my heart. That would really be a tragedy. So, when I have occasional feelings of sadness or despair, I work hard to turn that negative energy into a positive thing. It's like a miracle that has happened to my life. Maybe I can inspire other caregivers, and they will see they too can find new strength.

Martha immediately accepted her daughter's need for care resulting from the car accident. There were no right or wrong choices in this situation. Her husband didn't want a totally dependent child living with the family, yet Martha felt strongly about keeping her dependent daughter at home. Although she didn't share much about their marriage problems, it was obvious that Martha's intention of providing the necessary care for Janice at home contributed to an already failing marriage. I didn't encounter Martha after our original meeting, so I'm not aware if she engaged community services for help or requested occasional relief from neighbors, relatives, or friends, but I hope that she did.

Many people who take on the responsibility of being a family caregiver, who feel they can and should assume the total burden, run the risk of becoming overworked, run down, and vulnerable both physically and emotionally. The view that I can do it all isn't always wise, yet Martha was able to find joy and satisfaction in providing care for her daughter, Janice. Martha was able to turn her tears of sadness into gifts of self-confidence, love, and appreciation despite the challenges of her situation. Martha's story shows us that hope and determination can grow out of circumstances that are often viewed only as negative.

1. Do you work with or know family caregivers who have assumed the entire role of an around-the-clock caregiver? Why do you think they have made that decision? How have you been able to help them—perhaps by providing information or making connections?

2. Although Martha didn't talk about getting help from others, what stories can you share of neighbors and others who have graciously offered help and aided family caregivers in various ways?

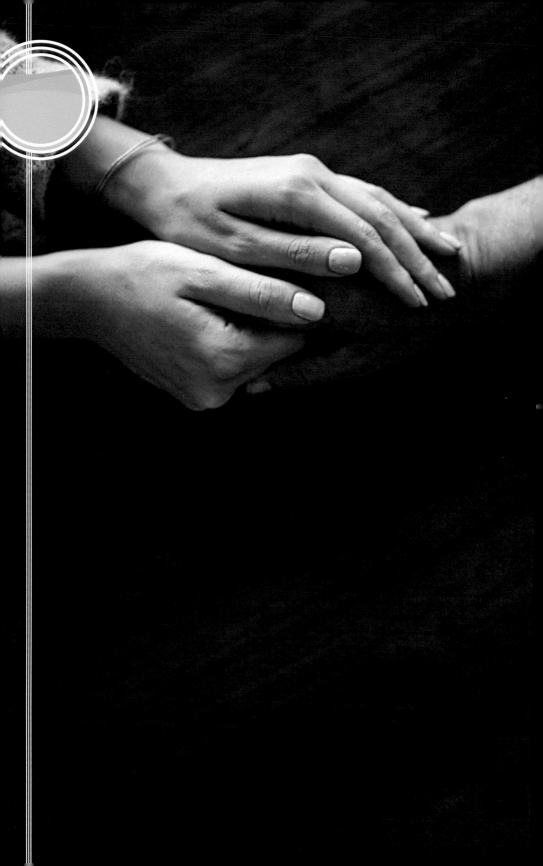

HERBERT

WE HAVE EACH OTHER

ALTHOUGH THE MAJORITY OF FAMILY CAREGIVERS IN THE country are women, many men have accepted the responsibility of primary caregiver. Herbert cares for his wife, Jill, who has Parkinson's disease, a degenerative spine, and other medical complications. The couple married young, and Jill's Parkinson's disease began during the first few months of their marriage. Jill now needs constant care. When Herbert goes to work, either Jill's mother or an aide is there to help until he gets home. Herbert says that through the experience of caregiving for his wife, he has become more sensitive to, and aware of, the needs of others. "I've had an opportunity to explore a side of myself that many men don't. I've learned a lot about expressing my emotions and my feelings." His deep sensitivity and vulnerability was evident in my conversation with Herbert. Here is the essence of his personal caregiving experience.

I live with a woman who has been progressively disabled by Parkinson's disease for nineteen years. I don't really know how I would handle this situation if it were me, but ask my wife. She's the real hero of our family. Her name is Jill, which means "blithe or youthful spirit," and that describes her exactly. She's got a twinkle in her eye, and she's my little leprechaun, my little Irishwoman. We laugh a lot. We have to remember to do that. There are always tears, but we joke through them. Every once in a while, when the clouds move aside, I get to see her again, the joyful one I married. That's what keeps me going. Her occasional smile is an anchor for me.

It's not life as I thought it would be or planned early in our marriage many years ago, but it's real life, and it's deeper than I ever thought it would or could be. There's an overall goal in my life greater than making it in business or acquiring material things. I can do all sorts of things in my life out there in the world, but when I walk in through the doors of my home, I totally take on the life with my wife. There can be tears at any moment of our day, and there often are. Yet, in the midst of the crying, the pain, the falling, and the stitches, there's real joy, and that for me is the fulfillment of my life.

I haven't any need to talk about my care of Jill publicly, but recently our local Caregiver Resource Center gave me an award for what they called my inspiring example of devoted and conscientious caregiving. I appreciated it a lot, but I didn't want to make a big deal of it. Yet it gave me an opportunity to tell something about what goes on in our home and what people who are family caregivers have an opportunity to learn. I wrote a little speech about that. Here's some of what I said.

> Imagine yourself disabled. Can't? Most of us cannot, because we are not. Those who are certainly know what it's like. They know well what it's like to wake up in the morning but not be able to get out of bed. They know the frustration of seeing their clothing hanging in the closet and aren't able to even

begin to dress themselves. They know what it's like to feel the call of nature but not be able to get themselves to the bathroom. They know what it's like to fall when they try to walk and not be able to protect themselves from being hurt. They know what it's like to drool but not be able to wipe it off without help. They know what it's like to wait and wait and wait. Wait until your caretaker gets you out of bed. Wait until your caregiver dresses you. Wait until your helper has time to take you to the bathroom, and then wait until they come back to get you. Continually waiting for someone else because you simply can't do anything yourself, nothing, ever.

Ask yourself, what if I get seriously sick? Dare I become disabled? Who will take care of me? How will I pay for my care? Who can I trust? Will my friends abandon me? Will I be a burden to my friends and family? Will my family stay by me and help me? How will I deal with the guilt of being a burden to everyone? What will happen to my children, my dreams, my plans, and my savings? Will I be put in some kind of institution if someone will not be able to care for me? Will I have any dignity left when another person dresses me, feeds me, bathes me, and wipes me?

That's what I said, but what's most important to me is that Jill and I know we have each other. This gives us each stability and predictability in how we live each day. It's one day at a time, yet our hope is for many good days. I always tell Jill that we're going to go through this together, whatever comes. I reach out and hold her, cradle her, and let her know that I'm here for her now and that I'll always be here with her.

When I transcribed the recording of my conversation with Herbert, there were tears in my eyes. The depth of his commitment, the love and partnership between Herbert and Jill, is a beautiful human connection to witness. Yes, Herbert has his work, other family connections, and generous neighbors. If I told their entire story it would be a whole book. Each of the stories of family caregivers in this book are only a few pieces of each of their complicated and busy lives. Yet each story touches on an attitude, action, or reaction to a loved one's illness and dependence, and very often a continuing deterioration of health and loss of independence.

In many of my conversations with family caregivers I've heard of their complicated days as they juggle the needs of husbands and wives, grown children, and young grandchildren, as well as commitments to jobs and other activities. Becoming a committed caregiver in the midst of already busy and complicated lives often leaves little time for a one-to-one relationship with the person in care. Herbert's story reminds us that we need to make these caring, loving relationships a priority. The pile of dirty dishes and the bed linen can wait, but the loved one in care needs us now.

1. When have you been in a situation where the task to be done took priority over the person who needed you just to be with him or her? How have you handled this? Did an incident or unexpected experience lead you to change your priorities?

2. Think of a family caregiver who might come to a new awareness and possibly change his or her priorities after hearing this story.

3. How can we lessen the constant pressure in our culture to get things done and be productive? How can we get away from the pressure of the "to do today" list?

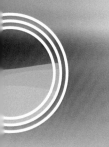

LOIS

A DIFFERENT PERSPECTIVE

THE 2014 UNITED STATES CENSUS TELLS US THERE ARE 76 MILLION baby boomers. Many of them are involved with caring for an elderly and frail parent. Very often parents live far from where their adult children have settled. Long-distance caregiving pre-sents many logistical challenges. Sometimes adult children make the decision to move closer to the parent; often, the more practical solution is to move the parent closer to the adult children. Either situation requires compromises, adjustments, and logistical and emotional challenges. Old resentments, suppressed anger, and feelings of childhood deprivation can add to the stress of the situation. Lois will tell you that it's never too late to heal old hurts, though. We talked about this when I came to visit her. We sat in her charming kitchen in a wooded residential area. Our conversation was about healing, not of the body but of the relationship between parent and child.

M y parents lived in Florida. My husband and I lived in the northern part of the country. After my father died my mother spent her time with her friends and her card games. Things seemed to be going normally until she developed uterine cancer. Even though it was a large tumor, the prognosis after surgery was good. But after about two years, they found a spot on her lung. The cancer had spread. She was sick and living alone in Florida. Many of her friends had either died or were moving away. I kept going back and forth to Florida to check on her. The stress and the constant travel exhausted me. One day I realized this arrangement just wasn't going to work. My husband and I began having conversations about the possibility of my mother moving closer to us.

I had always had a very difficult relationship with my mother. I could barely stand to be with her even one or two nights, and here I was thinking about bringing her to live close to me. I had spent a lifetime wanting a better relationship with my mother, but I had no clue how to fix it. We just couldn't communicate. As a child I once blurted out, "You never tell me you love me!" And she said, "That's not how we do it. I don't have to say it. Of course I love you." During my adolescence, our conversations became irrelevant or contentious. I left home, went to college, married, and embarked on raising my own family. Living in another city, I maintained a cordial but rather superficial relationship with my mother. Now the state of her health was changing everything.

My brothers were angry about the plan to move Mother. They couldn't believe I wanted to take her away from her friends and from the place where she had made her home in her retirement. However, they weren't the ones making the constant trips to Florida. That seemed to be the role of the only daughter. Also, I guess I secretly hoped that, living close to my mother, there might be a chance to work on a relationship that had disintegrated or maybe one that never really existed. I was hoping that this could be a chance to know this woman whom I had, for so much of my life, resented and certainly didn't understand. That, in fact, is exactly what happened.

I asked my mother how she felt about moving, and she almost immediately agreed that it would be good to live close to us. I looked for independent living situations near where I lived and found a great place she liked. To my surprise, she made immediate plans to move, and one month later Mother arrived, ready to set up a new life. At seventy-eight, she was a very independent woman; she made friends easily and played cards every day.

After a time we found that the cancer had spread. She trusted my husband and me to do the right thing for her. Like families often do in the face of a terminal disease, we desperately searched for a medical miracle to cure her cancer. But what happened was a healing instead of a cure, a healing of the relationship between my mother and me. The time she was with us gave me a chance to know a different mother, and she took the opportunity to finally get to know her daughter. Not until I became her caregiver did I realize how much we both needed each other. Building a genuine relationship with my mom during the two years she lived here was a mutual gift that grew from my sharing what life she had left and then participating in her dying.

I began to see another side of my mother. She knew the prognosis was not good, but she went through it all with a smile on her face. I saw her resiliency as she scarcely shed a tear over what she had left behind or what lay ahead. She poured herself into doing whatever she could to survive, and she did it with amazing style and grace. My mother showed me what it meant to truly live in the face of death.

I remember being amazed when, shortly after her arrival, I took her shopping for a winter coat. No basic black utilitarian number for her; she selected a bright red wool coat with a smashing black velvet beret. And each time she wore it, whether to a grueling chemotherapy treatment or someplace more pleasant, she lit up with a special joie de vivre that blew me away. I've kept that coat and have worn it each winter since she died. Each time I put it on, it's as if she has her arms around me giving me that warm hug I always craved.

Even when the red coat was out of season, she somehow remained cloaked in unfathomable optimism. She made new friends, took advantage of nearly every excursion offered at her new residence, and kept herself looking beautiful at all times. Our trip to buy a wig, in anticipation of her losing her hair as a result of chemotherapy, was colored by her sense of adventure about finding a new hairdo, not the dread of what was to come. I was on the verge of tears at the horror of what she, who was always so concerned about her appearance, would have to face. Yet she joked with the saleswoman and gently tried to prod me into considering a wig for myself so I wouldn't have to be bothered with my unruly natural curls in the summer humidity. It was a brave display of humor and courage.

The bleakness of her prognosis did not interfere with her determination to go on living for as long as she could. She loved to shop and tuned to cable TV shopping when she could no longer manage the shopping trips, or she'd thumb through catalogs and order herself occasional gifts. If her phone didn't ring, she simply picked it up and called me or someone else she knew to make plans. Her conversations were cheerful and upbeat. Even when she began to have periods of disorientation, she was aware of what was happening and could even laugh about them.

As her disabilities increased and she became less and less able to carry on independently, she gratefully and graciously welcomed the opportunity to have shifts of hired caretakers help her remain in her own apartment. They too became her friends, inspired by her quiet courage and her refusal to complain. I got to see resilience that I never knew my mother possessed.

When Mother was weak and tired, we would often sit together. Quiet was okay. Doing nothing was okay. Just being there with her, sitting quietly with her was healing. I learned about silence, about not needing to be doing something all the time. That was a special lesson that I was privileged to have learned, and I treasure it. She had a zest for life, and even in her illness she taught me how to take each day as a gift and simply live it, enjoy it. We never talked about what had happened to our relationship in the past. We just let it grow and change, and we both sensed a mutual acceptance—and love— emerging. We really got to know who each of us was, and we both really enjoyed every minute of our new connection.

We never had those heart-to-heart talks on the meaning of life that I had so often craved, but each time we greeted and parted, our hugs got tighter and longer. Early on I had begun saying to her, "I love you," and she immediately responded in kind. It was something I had desperately wanted to hear as a child. We exchanged those words in every phone call and every visit thereafter. They sustained both of us, and a connection I had never before felt grew and thrived. When she died in my arms, I whispered, "I love you," and I knew that she had heard me when it mattered, and I had heard her too.

The whole experience was a gift. Often you hear of people working so hard to heal rifts and misunderstandings between mother and daughter. Our situation was quite different. Just letting go of the old stuff allowed our transformation to happen. Suddenly she became a beautiful person, and I truly appreciated her. We began to enjoy every single moment we spent together. It was very precious.

Maybe people always have the opportunity to see things differently, but we just don't let ourselves understand that. Maybe a sense of urgency, when time is short, suddenly allows something like this to happen. I recall thinking that this horrible disease is killing my mother, and yet it's giving us the gift of a deep relationship we never would have had.

Her dying was profoundly moving and unforgettable. My children got to see their grandmother die with dignity and a sense of integrity. When she died, I felt a warmth and peacefulness envelop me. To actually be there with her was uplifting and wonderful. I never would have believed it. I think the greatest gift, my legacy, was that my negative, unconstructive relationship with my mother had been healed. I miss her still, so very much. She's alive to me in so many ways. It is a magical, mystical connection that I deeply treasure.

The experience with my mother has also enriched my relationship with my husband. Since her death, we've reorganized our priorities, slowed down together. We value our lives in a new way. We've really worked at it. In facing my mother's death, we've come to understand that everyone's life has a beginning and at some time an end. I'm an attorney, mainly in family law issues, and that keeps me extremely busy. I've recently made considerable changes and have begun to renurture myself. I'm working on saying no to more work, and my husband is doing the same. As my perspectives have evolved, my husband has also talked of wanting to change his pace and explore a life in the slow lane. Such changes have not been easy, but we're doing it. It is amazing to now have plans that I would have thought were impossible.

The experience with my mother started me on this new path. Suddenly her life ended, and it hit me. When you personally experience it, you get it. It's ironic that we learn more about life by learning about death, but I think that is true. We're learning not to let life run by us. I know that it's the real learning. For me, nothing will ever take that away.

I haven't seen a survey or study to back this up, but I've heard in many conversations over the years about women who have had issues with their mothers that resulted in negative feelings and distant relationships throughout their lives. Lois, who reluctantly offered to care for her mother nearby, received an unanticipated opportunity to heal their relationship, learn about themselves, and deepen their affection for each other. Their experience confirms that healing and learning about oneself are always options if we find the right path and dare to take it.

Lois talked about another big learning for herself. She realized that rather than constantly tending to tasks and instead sitting quietly with her mother and just being together was a rewarding experience for each of them. Our society encourages us to get things done, use our time constructively, and keep busy. Her caregiving experience opened her to possibilities for a change of pace in her life. There's no way of measuring the value of just being with someone, listening to what the person wants to say, expressing love for him or her, or maybe watching the birds together out of the nearest window. Spending relaxed time with the person in care may offer unexpected gifts in a relationship and an opportunity to see both the present and the future from a different perspective.

1. How often have you found your work and other family commitments have left little or no time to simply *be* with the person in your care? Share a personal story or one you've been told about that involves leaving the household tasks for later to focus on the one in your care.

2. Many women I've known personally and professionally have shared stories of healing in their mother-daughter relationship. Often it grew out of a caregiving experience with their mother. What stories can you tell about healing—from professional experience, a personal situation, or possibly both?

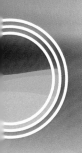

JEANNE

CELEBRATING THE LIFE WE'VE SHARED

THIS IS A STORY ABOUT A MOTHER AND A SON—NOT A FRAIL, elderly mother being cared for by a son, but a mother in her early fifties caring for a son diagnosed with AIDS. Jeanne was eager to tell me about her son, Michael, and his partner, Jim, with whom she shared the caregiving experience.

Jeanne is aware that many parent-child relationships have been shattered by AIDS. "I know too many people estranged from their living children. I hope my experience will encourage tolerance and understanding in families that have rejected a son who is sick or dying." Through her tears, Jeanne related her experience of pain and personal growth.

W̲e didn't know he had AIDS. My son, Michael, had gone into the hospital with a collapsed and infected lung. His white blood cell count was extremely low, so the doctors tested his immune system and found he had AIDS. He was told he probably had only a few months to live, but Michael survived another three years after that original diagnosis. During that time I spent about four to five hours every day with him. I'd work in the morning, then go to visit him and stay until his partner, Jim, came home. During the last six months of Michael's life, we brought hospice care into the house, because my son wanted to die at home. The doctor suggested that the amount of love around him from me, his family, and his partner helped him to live those additional three years. I knew my son really loved me, and I truly loved him.

Michael's illness took me down many different caregiving paths. The first six months of his illness were the hardest for me. I cried, raged, and actually had isolated periods of screaming. I'm a homeopathic practitioner of complementary medicine, with a specialty in alternative medicine. I couldn't find a way to help, even though I felt I knew how to help, both as a mother and a healer. But Michael resisted my help, which frustrated me, since he had always bragged about the work I did. He resisted my suggestions about diet, supplements, and homeopathy. I finally got him to try some Chinese formulas to build up his bone marrow, and he was better for a while. But as soon as he found out that it worked, he stopped. I realized then that my son might not have wanted to live. I believe a subconscious part of him—fighting a disease that has no cure—didn't want to be here. That was the hardest thing for me to accept.

Here was my beloved son, the one who'd promised that when I went to an old folks' home, he'd pull the hairs out of my chin so I didn't look silly. He was going to take care of me and read to me, and now he was the one who was dying. I felt a profound sense of abandonment and betrayal. I also experienced constant sadness and grief. You're not supposed to lose a child. I had to get to a spiritual place to give me the perspective I needed to learn. If you truly love someone, you have to honor what he or she wants to do. It doesn't have to be the way you want it; it doesn't have to make sense to you. You have to love them that much. I began to see clearly that I needed to learn how to celebrate the life he had, the man he was.

The time I spent with my dying son was probably the most beautiful and most painful period of my life. We shared an intimacy that, except for my husband, I've never shared with another person. During that time, my biggest challenge as a caregiver was to learn how to be present in the moment and to have no expectations. I spent so many hours with him. We would just hang out together. I'd sit by the bed, read, write, crochet, and watch TV. He'd wake up and look over at me and go back to sleep. Sometimes we talked for hours. We were totally honest about our deepest feelings. I believe that if someone knows they are going to die, it's important to help them validate the life they've had. Toward the end, Michael and I reviewed his life, and doing that together gave purpose and meaning to a lot of what he had done. It helped me let go and to be more accepting of the reality of his condition. I had the choice to fall apart or to see how dealing with the death of my child could teach me to become stronger.

The experience of Michael's dying taught me to appreciate the gift of what you have in front of you, instead of crying about what you are not going to have. I learned to just live in this moment. And if you truly live that way, you are not losing the person. They're here, and you're here. There was nothing my son and I didn't say to each other. We discussed it all. I don't regret the tragedy of the way he died—how long it was. I feel blessed I had the time with him that I did. Others lose someone in a second. I had this time to be with him. It was truly beautiful.

I recall one night when I was watching television, and Larry King was interviewing former Los Angeles Dodgers manager Tommy Lasorda, who had lost his son when he was only thirty. Larry King asked him, "How did you get through that? Where is the meaning in the loss of a child?" And Tommy said, "I look at it this way. If God came down and stood in front of me and said, 'Tommy, I've got a deal for you. I'm going to give you this incredible kid. But you'll only have him for thirty years. What do you want to do?'" Tommy Lasorda said, "I would do it all again." And I agree.

I have all those memories of the child and the man he became, and you cannot be sorry for it. What I mean is that I realized what a gift I had. I've learned to be more attentive to those I love now. Life is fragile, and you can lose anyone at any moment. They need to know you love them, and you need to allow them to love you. Let them in. Make time. I truly appreciate that I was blessed. We had an unconditional love together.

I believe you need to continue to celebrate the life of a loved one who has died. I used to bring Michael sunflowers. He was like sunshine, his face like a sunflower. Once a week I'd bring a new bouquet of sunflowers. He'd beam when I entered the room. So now on his birthday, and also on the anniversary of the evening of his death, each of us in our close family takes a sunflower to the pier at the water near where we live. We quietly remember Michael in our own way and drop our sunflowers into the ocean in memory, in love. It's our celebration of a life, of Michael's life.

I had this conversation with Jeanne several years ago. Those were the days when people were just beginning to understand HIV and AIDS. Now early diagnosis doesn't offer a cure, but medications allow years of an active life.

Michael knew he was dying before his mother Jeanne was ready to accept that reality. He wasn't interested in prolonging his dependent lifestyle. Before Jeanne could come to accept the reality of her son's situation, she was unable to take any pleasure and satisfaction in sharing each day with her son. Learning to live in the moment totally changed that.

The longer each of us lives, we face the reality that illness, accidents, limitations, and dependency are possible. To be open to the reality of a situation and accept it, as Jeanne's story illustrates, can offer unexpected enjoyment and deepening of each encounter. Memories can be loving and joyous as we commemorate a loved one who has passed on. Of course, we mourn, but we can also celebrate the life we've shared.

1. When have you been involved in a situation where the person in care has given up treatments and medications, knowing that the outcome will be an end to his or her life? How have individuals in that family responded? What have you learned from such an experience and from the reactions of others?

2. Jeanne's story offers a unique perspective of a parent caring for an adult child who will predecease her. Have you dealt with such a circumstance either personally or professionally? What unique challenges have you faced in dealing with this?

3. Michael's life is celebrated in personal and unique ways, such as the sunflower ceremony. What experiences have you had with commemorative events or other rituals that keep the departed person's memory alive?

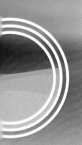

ELBERT

SHE WENT EVERYWHERE WITH ME

SERVING AS A CAREGIVER TO A LOVED ONE WITH ALZHEIMER'S disease or any condition of mental deterioration can be a heart-wrenching, stressful, and confusing experience. To maintain a relationship of dignity and respect in the face of the personality and behavioral changes that often come with such illness is an enormous challenge. Elbert Cole is a Methodist minister but no longer the head of a congregation. When Elbert Cole's wife, Virginia, was diagnosed with Alzheimer's, he and their adult children devised a personal plan of caregiving that ultimately offered great rewards. As a family, they discussed her present condition and the projected decline, divided up responsibilities, and made plans to live as normally as possible. Virginia lived for seventeen years with Alzheimer's. Elbert Cole talked with me about her life and her death.

Before Virginia was diagnosed, I saw symptoms that things were not right. Early on we met as a family—my two adult children and my wife, Virginia, too. At this point, the deterioration was just beginning. Our son, who is a scientist, explored the latest research on Alzheimer's to see if there was any chance of hope or relief. If there was, we wanted to know about it. But we knew that if we really wanted to be helpful, we needed to pursue not the dream of a cure but the path of caregiving.

We dedicated ourselves to finding ways of keeping Virginia looking well dressed and fashionable. My daughter took that on. Virginia and I negotiated a new partnership, and I decided she would go everywhere with me. I made no apologies and asked no permission. I pulled up a chair at board tables and anywhere else I needed to go, and she just sat there and enjoyed the whole proceeding. Her task was simply to be with me, to enjoy.

Instead of withdrawing from life and feeling that I should be ashamed, I felt proud of Virginia. I assumed that if people couldn't accept her condition, then they, not she, had the problem. I coached the children so they wouldn't worry if their mother was quiet when they called. It only meant that she was listening carefully to every word they were sharing with her. I advised them to keep on talking normally. Virginia would just sit and smile. She knew that at the other end of the phone was somebody who loved her.

To feel good about themselves, everyone needs to know they're loved and respected. They also need to feel secure, to be included and not alienated or marginalized, to celebrate the joy of life, and to feel needed. Having Alzheimer's doesn't change such things. When you're dealing with someone who seems to be on a whole different level, a simple childlike level, it can become too easy to see that person as inferior. If you don't respect the other person as someone who still has something to contribute, then you can too easily begin treating her like a *thing,* an object that must be dressed and fed rather than a person with whom you can share life.

Of course, it isn't always easy to maintain such respect, but if we prematurely make other people's decisions and dominate them, we can shut them off from their ideas or input for planning their own lives. It's a balance to allow freedom and yet take on the responsibility of being a caregiver and making life as good as possible for the other person.

Virginia was different from many other people who have Alzheimer's. She was quiet, never demanding, always gracious and appreciative of what was done for her. It's amazing that she retained that capacity, given what you read in the literature and hear about other situations. For me, for us as a family, she was never a burden. I tried to keep Virginia connected to the world and stimulated. She had a deep interest in art, so we often went to museums. We walked through shopping centers to look at things. And she loved to talk with children. At times, of course, she'd do inappropriate things, like pat a man's backside or reach for a woman's purse or go over to children she didn't know and pat their heads. But I never felt ashamed of Virginia; I never felt apologetic. I did occasionally have a wistful thought about how nice it would be if she (and we) had better years ahead, but on the other hand, we made the most of what we had.

We shared a lot. I loved traveling with her, spending time with her, and taking her with me to meetings and speeches.

And we laughed together. Humor is so important in life. It's healing. It's relaxing. It lightens things up, and it keeps you out of self-pity. When you're dealing with dementia, you're dealing with a world of fantasy and imagination, and there's richness and beauty in such places. I don't think it should be thought of as bad. Sure, somebody needs to be around who knows where the real world is, but life can still be good for the person living partly in another reality.

Caregiving must never become an unmanageable burden. If it does, it's wrong, and the price you pay will be too great. A person who has the responsibility to coordinate the care of a loved one has to know what he can handle and what he can't. There need be no guilt involved in recognizing limits. You do what you need to do. Some people can't handle or don't choose to handle the burdens, frustrations, and adjustments. In my situation our family shared those challenges and reaped the rewards. Our whole family felt that Virginia continued to teach us so much all the way to the end. We discovered that all kinds of rewards come, some quietly and unexpectedly. Virginia taught us how to slow down a bit. She taught us a kind of a peace and a quiet courage. We all learned lessons from her. When you live with someone acting out her life with increasing limitations, you can't help but begin to rethink your own life and what's really important.

Once, when Virginia was quite weary, I decided I wouldn't take her along for my speech that evening. When I came back, she was lying on top of the bed with the light on, asleep. I leaned over, and she awoke with a childlike smile on her face, knowing that her friend had come home.

The next morning, as I was giving her a shower, she began to hyperventilate, and I knew that her life was ending. She was obviously under some strain. So I put her back on the bed and sat on the edge of the bed for two hours just watching her, talking to her about our history and our children and everything we had accomplished in our lives together. And I told her how courageous I thought she had been and what a wonderful wife and mother she had been. And she just laid there and watched me and smiled, and listened and listened and listened. And then finally she had no strength left, and the life just left her body.

I took her in my arms and started to recite the Twenty-third Psalm. I must admit, because of my emotion and tears, I skipped about every other line. I am grateful that we had this time of privacy and that she died in peace.

With all the stories of the difficulties of mental illness, it's easy to lose sight of the tenderness that people share with loved ones. For me, being able to celebrate the tenderness, talk about it, affirm it, and say *that's* what I remember became a real gift. I think it was a gift for Virginia too. We'd had fifty-four years of marriage. Her illness extended over seventeen of those years. I've not lingered much on what could have been. I know how wonderful it was that we continued to journey together, and maybe that was my greatest gift of all.

There aren't any right or wrong answers for a family choosing how to publicly deal with a family member's diminished and changed behavior, as each situation is very different. Families must make these decisions by honestly assessing the situation and their own opinions and fears. In some situations, the person with such changes may offer some input. Elbert's thoughts and actions as his wife's Alzheimer's progressed were different from many other people's in such situations. As Virginia was reasonably quiet and manageable, he took her along to meetings and other gatherings so she could have the comfort of being with him and feeling included.

I suspect that including the person with progressive dementia most often would not be comfortable or appropriate for either the patient or the group asked to receive her, especially for someone with Alzheimer's who exhibited unsociable behaviors. Some families are uncomfortable and don't want to be publicly associated with a person in their family who has dementia. They feel embarrassed when a family member exhibits erratic behaviors. However, I believe that if a person with dementia does not exhibit behavior that disrupts and distracts others, he or she could be included in a large family event or at public get-togethers.

Many Americans are living longer these days—into their late eighties, nineties, and even over one hundred. Memory losses and changes often accompany aging minds, and tolerance and understanding need to be exercised by both them and their families.

1. **Have you lived with or dealt personally or professionally with a person with memory loss? What stories can you share that might offer some insight into decisions about going out in public?**

2. **If you have dealt with a person experiencing memory loss, with someone who has received a diagnosis of dementia, or with family members caring for a loved one with memory problems, what practical strategies have you used to help him or her maintain as much independence as possible?**

3. **How can family members learn to become patient and understanding of the insecurity often felt by someone with memory deterioration?**

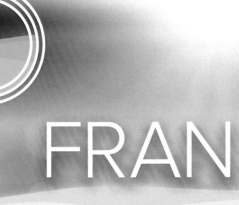

FRAN

FINDING MY WAY TO HEAL

"I'M FIFTY-SIX NOW," FRAN TOLD ME AS WE BEGAN OUR CONVER-
sation. "It's about time I let go of the pain and the sadness and
move on." She was talking about an old emotional wound, one
that wasn't healed before her father died. I think it's important
to share her story, because it reminds us that not being able to
repair a damaged relationship with a dying parent can profoundly
affect a surviving child's life. Fran talked openly about her experience in the hope that her story will help others.

It was ten years ago that my dad died. I came into my caregiving role unexpectedly. I was living in Japan and teaching English as a second language. I had no idea that my dad was sick. One day, out of the blue, I got a call from my aunt telling me that my dad had had a lung biopsy and had been diagnosed with advanced lung cancer. She told me to come home quickly, so I packed up and left Japan. My dad lived only a couple of weeks after my arrival.

Dad insisted on being at home those last few weeks. He was eighty years old and in a great deal of pain, and he seemed ready to get out of this world as quickly as possible. To him, being in a hospital and getting any treatment only prolonged the inevitable. He didn't want strangers in his house. He was fearful that someone coming in to help might be a medical person sent to prolong his life. He was suspicious of everything, even ordinary pain medication.

I didn't know how to care for a dying person, and I didn't know anyone in the community to ask for help. I tried to convince Dad to let hospice come to the house, but he absolutely refused. The most difficult thing for me was facing this all alone. I wasn't emotionally ready to tackle the caregiver role and not at all prepared psychologically for dealing with my father. There were many unresolved issues between us. The unsatisfying quality of those few weeks we spent together as he was dying still hangs over me. It's sad that both my dad's and my experience of those last days of his life couldn't have been a time of reconciliation and healing.

My father and I had spent our lives butting heads. As a child and a teenager, I didn't understand him, and he didn't understand me. Layers of anger and hurt had built up between us. I had been raised in a home where we didn't talk about things, certainly never about emotions. My father's life was colored by many losses, and I now understand how this shaped who he was. His mother died by suicide when he was fifteen, and he was sent away to military school. His father died of a heart attack soon after I was born. My mother died a few years later. Dad remarried quickly after my mother's death, and his second wife died within a year. I remember thinking that maybe if I had a child, if I made my dad a grandfather, some of the hurt would heal. So I got pregnant and found in the middle of my term that I had a very rare form of cancer that you get only when you are pregnant, choriocarcinoma. The placenta reproduces cells incorrectly and kills the fetus. For me, it was a life-threatening illness. My recovery was long and slow.

That my dad wanted me to come and be with him in his last days, and that I didn't hesitate to come, might indicate we both wanted some healing of our relationship. It was sad that we didn't know how to make that happen. He didn't want me to see him as a sick and dying old man, and I had never been around death and didn't know how to deal with it. At the time, I didn't know how to deal with the residual anger that had piled up between us all those years, so I wasn't able to reach out. Neither of us could talk to each other in a meaningful way.

My dad died without our saying good-bye to each other. In spite of it all, I believe we both knew that we loved each other. Sadly, an incredible silence hung between us. I don't remember even touching him. The healing that might have been possible never happened. To have my dad die without any reconciliation between us has been a heavy emotional road for me to travel these ten years since his death.

In recent years some healing has come for me through a new understanding of who he was and why he reacted to me as he did throughout his life. I discovered that his personal life was full of loss. That gave me some understanding of his inability to connect with people. I can remember him now with tenderness and a loving feeling that I could never experience when he was alive.

After my father's death I felt strongly that I had to find a different career for myself. Teaching English and living in a foreign country no longer felt right for me. I craved a new direction that included work that touched my heart and deepened my feelings. I needed work that would help me heal and allow me to help others. One day a friend came to talk to me about an idea for a project she wanted to create: a series of workshops to help her deal with the death of her mother and for others who have lost their parents. It was as if an inner voice said, "This is what you've been looking for."

Together we created a series of workshops and groups called Healing Hearts. Our work is different from other grief support groups in that we assist only people who are having difficulties dealing with the death of a parent. Many people we work with are older, and it may have been many years since their loss. Suddenly the sadness, the guilt, and the grief can resurface, as mine did, which isn't unusual. I feel that in many ways what I'm doing with my life now is exactly what I should be doing. My personal history of loss provides me with a way to help others with their issues surrounding the loss of a parent.

What have I learned from all this? Well, I've learned that you can heal a relationship with a parent even after his or her death. I've learned that if people experience continual loss, it affects their life and the lives of those around them profoundly. I'm gratified that I can help other people face feelings similar to what I've faced, and that I can heal myself by helping them. Walking with other people through their journey helps me realize that it's never too late, and that we shouldn't close the door to any opportunity for change and growth. Healing and change is an opportunity that appears from an unexpected place. This is what my life purpose is.

Healing Hearts is an enterprise that will never make us rich. But that really doesn't matter. It's not the reason I'm doing this. If it ever becomes work that puts making money first, then I'll know it's time for me to get out. For me, what I'm doing is life affirming, heart centered, and spiritually fulfilling.

My relationship with my own mother was difficult. But my opinion, which has evolved over the more than twenty years since she died, is that there are many ways to heal unfinished business with a mother or father who is no longer with us. Our relationship with them—both the interactions that have helped us grow in positive ways and those that have left us with regrets, limitations, and the need for closure—is inside us.

Each situation is different, and very personal, so I offer no secret formula for healing. Many who work at forgiving a parent may also need to forgive themselves for keeping the negative stuff alive inside. I encourage adult children who are left with unresolved parent issues to seek support and help. Therapists, counselors, friends, and others can help that healing happen. Whenever we're honestly ready to change a lifetime pattern, when we're ready to take it all on, it's the right time.

Healing demands emptying out, removing self-built barriers, letting go of ingrained responses, and finding whatever path can bring change and healing. Changes often come in small pieces, one hurdle at a time. Finding the freedom to embrace ourselves without those old constraints might well be labeled a gift of caregiving for the caregiver.

1. What experience with your parent are you willing to work at resolving, or have you already been able to heal?

2. What experience have you had with a friend or relative who is burdened by regrets, guilt, and other burdens linked to a relationship with a now deceased parent? How have you been able to help others find a resolution to the pain they're carrying?

3. What new challenges has Fran's story brought up for you personally or professionally? How might her experience offer you a new direction to pursue in your life or with a client?

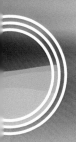

LIZ AND DAVE
IT CHANGED EVERYTHING

I ARRIVED AT LIZ AND DAVE'S HOME JUST AS SOME FRIENDS WHO had joined them for Sunday night supper were leaving. Liz and Dave had explained to me beforehand that their lives were too busy, their energy too committed to family matters, to make time during the day for an appointment with me. They suggested I come over in the evening after their daughters had gone to bed. At the end of a long day, somehow Liz and Dave pulled together the energy to tell me their story. They have three daughters. Two are typical girls in their teens. Their youngest daughter, Shoshi, who had just turned eleven, has a neurological disorder called Rett syndrome. Our conversation revealed a story of deep love, dedication, and commitment. Because Liz and Dave's opinions and answers to my questions were similar, I've combined them here into a single voice. Here's their story in their words.

Y ou've got your life and a family, and then something un-expected hits, and all the pieces fall to the ground like children's blocks. We knew quite early on that some-thing was not right, but even the most experienced doctors hadn't suspected Rett syndrome, because it is so rare. One neu-rologist finally diagnosed Shoshi as having Rett syndrome and said, "I'm so sorry to tell you that this child will not live past ten, and you will not be able to take care of her because she will self-mutilate," and on and on. This doctor turned our world upside down.

Kids with Rett syndrome are born seemingly normal, but be-tween the ages of one and two they lose skills they have just be-gun to develop, like speech, the ability to walk, and other motor and coordination skills. Shoshi first lost the use of her hands and developed a movement that looks like hand washing or clapping. She has a hand-to-mouth movement that she can't stop. It's re-petitive and constant. Her major handicap is the lack of motor skills. For example, Shoshi may want to look left and will instead look right. Many who have Rett syndrome cry in terror night af-ter night. When Shoshi screamed through the night, we couldn't find anything to soothe her. It was very, very difficult.

We've made the decision to care for Shoshi at home. She goes to a special school that can handle her needs for total care. In the summer, she goes to a camp program. Years ago, there would have been no way for us to do this. We are fortunate to live in a county that has many services, many agencies to deal with all kinds of special needs. We're so grateful to be in touch with all the advantages and services around us. We live in a dense, well-to-do metropolitan area, but if we were in a rural setting, we'd have far fewer advantages and services available to us. Still, we are constantly challenged to find the right education and therapy.

You ask what Shoshi can do. She can smile, hug, walk, eat if fed, and listen to us when we read or tell a story—but she's passive. We try to understand what it must be like for her, not being able to communicate or use her hands, not being able to say she is cold or hungry or in pain. If it were one of us, I think we'd just close up shop and check out of this world. What would be the point? Yet, despite all that she lives with, Shoshi keeps plugging along. She doesn't give up. A few weeks ago, we were in the hospital with her, and although she was drugged, she was strong and fighting to come back to her world. Her desire to belong in this world is very strong. She gives us the message that she not only wants to belong but she also has something to contribute. And that very often drives us. If she is willing to push, who are we to give up?

We believe that Shoshi and other children with Rett syndrome know and understand more than they can express, but measuring IQ is impossible. Neurologists claim that Rett syndrome is a developmental disorder and that once certain skills are lost, the deterioration will plateau. Yet, her medical issues are becoming more severe and pronounced. Things don't get better or even stay the same for Shoshi. It's been heartbreaking to watch our daughter progressively lose skills. This is something we continually deal with. Our world has caved in. To deal with this, we've had to pick up and build a new way to think and live.

We've learned a huge amount about patience and the wonderful gift of time. When we're with Shoshi, it is like being in a timeless zone. Last spring we went walking in a garden. We debated about letting her walk or not. We decided it didn't matter how long it took. So we walked, and she got tired and sat down on the pavement and just gazed and seemed delighted. We started talking about how we had scheduled ourselves on that walk. First, we needed to see this and then that and then go over there and not miss that. It was Shoshi who reminded us to just step back and enjoy the moment. She looked at the garden and after a short time fell asleep, and we had to just sit there. What a gift not to have a schedule, not to even look at a watch. Time didn't matter. We observed other families running around, and we sat there, and we both realized that this is such peace. We could look at the situation one way and say how sad it is, but we've learned to look at it all another way and see the gift.

We appreciate that we have gained so much from what we've learned because of our daughter's situation. We've become more conscious of the words we speak, to weigh them and consider the impact of what we say. Shoshi cannot speak at all, and at times we who have the gift of speech are guilty of misusing it. We thought about that recently when the spring was very wet and the water table was high, and our backyard and the yards of our neighbors were swamped. Some ugly, nasty language was exchanged between neighbors who blamed one another for the mud and mess draining into their yard because of the slope between houses. We are given the ability to speak, and what we learn from Shoshi is that this gift is not to be abused.

There are gifts that Shoshi is able to give to others at her special school. In kindergarten a troublemaker boy for some reason took a liking to Shoshi. The teacher decided to use Shoshi to modify his behavior. She told the boy that if he didn't hit anyone and if he did his assignment, he could have ten special minutes with Shoshi. And by gosh, he did his work and behaved. I guess he really wanted to be with her. Shoshi turned this kid into a kinder soul. And things like this keep going on. A group of teens helps us out on some weekends and evenings. A few of these kids are thinking about careers in special education based on their connection with Shoshi. Something about her gives a special meaning to people. It's profound. She teaches without words. Her spirit speaks loudly.

Shoshi attends a summer camp that has a program for kids with special needs. One day a little boy at the camp caught my eye. He was a sweet kid, a gentle soul. Every morning he chose to be with Shoshi. He wanted to push her stroller. He seemed to enjoy being with her so much. When he finally made the connection that Liz was her mother, he said, "Oh, you're Shoshi's mom. You are so lucky!" That took us completely by surprise. Usually from adults we hear Shoshi is lucky to have us. Yet, somehow, kids are happy to be with her. We marvel at this.

One of the hardest things about being a parent to a handicapped child is trying to maintain a normal life for the others in the family. We're a team, a unit. It's important for us to give the message to our other girls that they are special, too. We have three girls, and we believe that our energy as parents should be divided equally between each, although that always requires a little less sleep and a little more pushing to fit it all in. But no matter how preoccupied we get, we don't forget about the other kids. I recall one time last year when our daughter Chava asked if her mother could lead the girls' choir in her school. Our first response was to say, "Of course not; there isn't time to do that." But the second response was, "How could we possibly say no?" It wouldn't be fair. If our daughter Nomi is playing in a basketball game, for instance, we might not want to pack Shoshi up and make the effort to attend, but we know we must do it for Nomi.

When we talk to families whose child has recently been diagnosed with Rett syndrome, we suggest they take it a step at a time. Listening to them can bring tears to our eyes when we get off the phone. But we can't say much to the new families. We listen, we answer questions, but they'll have to learn the insights and lessons for themselves. It doesn't seem right to tell them what may be down the path. Look at now, we say. The point is, you plan for the future, but you live one day at a time. It gets you through. When we have a good day with Shoshi, we feel enormous gratitude.

With a handicapped child, there's no finality. The bad times don't end; it's a continual process. For us there's always deep, deep sorrow and often anger, and we suffer endless grief. You can be doing something like driving or shopping, and all of a sudden you feel hot tears behind your eyes. And sometimes we get mad at God. God is supposed to be compassionate, the healer of the sick, yet Shoshi elicits compassion in others. So maybe that's how we should interpret God, as the spirit of compassion.

We know we don't get enough sleep or physical exercise, and the emotional strain is constant. But we're blessed with many special friends who are part of our journey and our lives. We're always there for each other, and that's enormously important. We often hear of families who find support from their religion, but at this time we struggle with what that really means for us. We find strength from our other two daughters, and curiously, strength from Shoshi too.

We've gotten many comforting thoughts from Rabbi Kushner's book *When Bad Things Happen to Good People,* such as the notion that through people like Shoshi, godliness comes as a gift to all of us. But we'd trade it in a heartbeat for a little girl who could braid her own hair and do normal things. We often wonder at whose expense these lessons are being taught.

Perhaps someday we'll understand. But we would hope that there are more compassionate ways to learn these lessons that are not so tough on her.

For a young girl who has had so many things taken away from her, Shoshi shows a resilience that is special and rare. When we look at her, we can't help but marvel at the power of a smile! She can look right into your soul. We sense what she's thinking much of the time, but sometimes we can't, and we'll say, "Shoshi, we know you're telling us something, but we just don't understand." She's the patient one. She'll wait until we catch on.

We've shared with you the God wrestling that we constantly go through, yet we want you to know that for us, Shoshi is a bundle of love. We're both very proud of her. We like to take her places, even though every time we take her somewhere people stare. Sometimes things like this can pull families apart. Not us. We know we're in this together for the long haul.

Every time I share this story I feel great compassion and empathy for Shoshi's loving family. I've thought a lot about what life learning might result from a story so different from many of ours in almost every way. Yet, my experience continues to validate that a story not at all like our own can teach us new awareness and a different way of seeing some of our own issues.

Shoshi's parents commented that on learning of their daughter's diagnosis of Rett syndrome, their world might have totally caved in. Yet their sharing revealed how deciding to look at it as a gift delivered inside this tragedy changed everything, the way they now live their lives and what they continue to learn.

I was pleased to hear Liz and Dave talk about their other daughters and their continuing efforts to maintain a normal home life for them. No matter how long or difficult their day was, they made the effort to give each of their girls the attention they need, helping with their studies and outside activities and continuing to nurture total family sharing.

We so often hear variations of the phrase "We live one day at a time." When they said it in our conversation, they quickly added that although that was true, they continued to plan for the future. Each of us has hopes and plans for our futures, yet life often brings uncertainties. This story reminds us that how we choose to deal with our challenges shapes each of our lives.

1. **What challenges, losses, or burdens that have come into your life or the life of friends or clients have presented a life-changing, continuing obligation? Share a story about an event that could easily be viewed as hopeless and yet resulted in positive personal growth.**

2. **What changes in family involvements have you experienced or learned about from the *wholeness* of a caregiving situation—from the fact that a caregiving situation involves the entire family? Please share a story from your experience.**

3. **Whether an experience is labeled religious, spiritual, or mysterious, we all have heard of situations that are unexplainable, like the attraction of so many children to Shoshi. What stories can you share about a relationship or occurrence that is not easily understood? What have you learned from such situations? What has been your reaction to the story of Shoshi and her parents? Has it influenced your thinking in a meaningful way?**

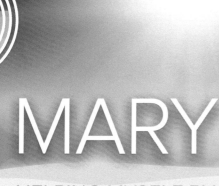

MARY

HELPING MYSELF BY HELPING OTHERS

MARY IS RETIRED AND LIVES ALONE. SHE WAS WIDOWED AT A young age, raised her family, and has generally led a life she'd label ordinary. Mary volunteers for a local hospice group and has discovered that there's nothing ordinary about the caring visits she makes to those who are sick and dying. There are hospice volunteer caregivers in big cities and small towns all over the United States. Each volunteer has his or her own reasons for doing this work; each has his or her individual experiences to share. Mary can tell only her story, but the rewards she finds in visiting the sick and dying aren't so different from those found by other volunteers. Mary is soft-spoken, modest, and friendly. She was seventy-two years old at the time of this interview. Our conversation began with her telling me a little about her younger years.

At the age of thirty-six I had two children and was expecting a third. That summer my husband wasn't feeling at all well. One doctor said it was ulcers, but another suspected stomach cancer, and that's what it turned out to be. First, they gave him cobalt treatments to shrink the tumors, and then they operated. They knew he wasn't going to fully recover after that. He came home from the hospital, and for the short time he lived I took care of him. My sister came out from New Jersey to help me with the three children, as I'd had the baby by then. Without my sister, I couldn't have managed. The day after I came home from the hospital after having the baby, my husband went back in, and they tried chemotherapy. That treatment was very new then. They knew he wouldn't make it, but they were determined to try everything. He was so young when he died.

Some months later, I went to work in the same hospital as a volunteer. I wanted to be able to walk by the hospital and not feel lost and sad. To start healing myself, I made myself go into the room my husband had been in. After a couple of years I gave up the volunteering, because I had to go back to work. It took me a long time to know that I could go on, to understand that I could find ways to have happiness in my life.

I was a teacher for many years, then I worked at the post office before taking retirement. That's when the work I'm doing now began. I started working with hospice. A friend of mine, a nurse, told me they needed volunteers badly. I told her I didn't know anything about medicine. And she told me, "Hospice isn't about medicine, hospice is about caring."

I went through a hospice training program, and one day I got a phone call and was asked if I'd like to visit an older woman who was dying of breast cancer. They needed someone just to sit and visit with her a few times a week. I rang her doorbell, went in, sat down, and then realized I really didn't know what to do or say. Finally I said, "Look, if you want to talk, I'd be happy to have a conversation with you. If you don't feel like talking, let me sit here and just be with you, okay?" We shared both silent times and deep conversations, and in the months before she passed away, we became close friends. During the years I've worked with hospice, I've made friends with many people who were dying. That's what hospice volunteers do.

One time I was assigned a lady in her midfifties who was dying of colon cancer. The doctor said she probably wouldn't live more than six months. On my first visit I didn't like her much. She was so angry that she was dying that talking with her was almost impossible. She was more difficult to be with than anyone I had ever visited before. The miracle was that we eventually became as close as sisters. We were of different lifestyles and very different temperaments. Yet our relationship worked for some unknown reason. I don't have patience in many situations, but in so many hospice visits I've made over the years I seem to have endless patience.

We talked about everything. She told me about her past, her husband, her family, her experiences. And we laughed together a lot. I spend a lot of time at her house, and the relationship we developed was wonderful. I know I gave her a great deal as a friend, and I got a great deal back: warmth, love, and appreciation, from both her and her husband. Her husband couldn't handle her illness and periodically had to leave for three or four days. I moved in when he was gone. She lasted a year and a half, much longer than the doctors predicted. I was with her when she died. She was a special person.

What I discovered in my hospice work was that I can give many who are ill and dying what they need, and it doesn't take anything away from me. So many of these people have hard struggles. Some are paralyzed; others can't talk or feed themselves. My visits give them some happiness, and actually, contact with them gives me back more than I give. People tell me that they could never be with people who are dying, and they wonder how I do this work. But for me, getting to know each person is a special and rewarding experience.

I'm doing something I didn't know I could do, and I'm really doing it well. I sincerely feel love for each person I get to know in my hospice visits. I tell them that they're loved, that they're cared for. When one of my new friends dies, I know that I've made a real difference in their last days. I guess what I do is help people die. I don't mean that in a bad way. What I'm saying is that I make their dying easier for them and their last days less lonely. When my time comes, I hope I have a hospice volunteer like me around.

––––––––––––––––

Over the years since I talked with Mary, I've become very familiar with what hospice offers. They've spread throughout the country since that time, although the agencies define for themselves what services they offer. Each hospice service trains its volunteers to be sensitive to the personal thoughts and opinions of the families being served. It's not unusual that close friendships between hospice workers and clients grow and thrive.

I've heard stories about how some families don't want hospice workers around, because they assume that means the death of the person in care is imminent. This isn't necessarily true. Yes, the patient has an illness he or she will not recover from, but a hospice worker can be a new friend who listens to the person the worker is assigned to visit. A hospice volunteer brings friendship and comfort to both a person in care and that person's family. The volunteer is an additional sensitive and understanding friend whose comfort, companionship, and caring is a gift.

1. Have you been in a caregiving situation when a hospice volunteer has visited and seen how his or her presence has benefited family members and the person in care? What stories have you heard from others about hospice volunteers?

2. If you are interested in volunteering with a hospice group in your community, consider reaching out to your local hospital or aging agency.

PEG

THE MOMENT EVERYTHING CHANGED

PEG AND I KNEW EACH OTHER IN OUR "CAREFREE YEARS." WE worked together at National Public Radio in Washington, DC. We were both single and totally preoccupied with our exciting and stimulating jobs. We were somewhat oblivious to the problems and challenges we might face as our lives become more complicated. Eventually Peg married her boyfriend, Rich, had a son, and two years later was pregnant again. Not long ago I had an opportunity to spend the day with Peg to catch up on the years we'd been out of touch. Peg talked about the birth of her daughter, Kate, who was born with a rare genetic defect called CHARGE syndrome. Kate is ten years old now. Peg's tale has no last chapter. It's an ongoing story.

W hen I was pregnant with Kate, I had no idea anything was wrong. The birth of my son had been easy. I figured Kate's birth would be fine too. I went into labor five and a half weeks early. At the hospital I was losing blood, so the doctors did an emergency caesarean section. It was a hard birth. I almost didn't make it. That was the day my husband's and my life as we knew it, and thought it would be, ended.

Most people don't know much about the genetic malady CHARGE that our daughter, Kate, was born with. Why bother going into it? It's such a long song and dance. When people ask what's wrong with Kate, I tell them that I'll explain it to them after they meet her or they'll expect to see a monster. I want to show them that she's a great kid.

The name CHARGE syndrome uses an acronym for the different parts of the body in which abnormalities appear. *C* stands for coloboma, a structure in the eye. *H* is for heart defects; *A*, for atresia of the choanae, blockage of the nasal passage; *R*, for retardation of growth and development; *G*, for genital and urinary abnormalities; and *E*, for ear abnormalities or hearing loss or both. They tell me that the genetic defect occurred about thirty-five days into the pregnancy. It's very rare, and hardly anything is known about it. Up until about fifteen years ago most of the babies with CHARGE syndrome didn't survive birth.

Kate's ears are malformed and abnormal. She's been tested as moderately to severely deaf. Kate does have some hearing on one side, and if she would wear a hearing aid, which she won't, she could hear some. Her nasal passages are blocked with bone. She has a couple of minor heart problems. She's considered legally blind, but thankfully she does have some vision. She doesn't look at people's faces, but she doesn't walk into things. Somehow she manages. Her esophagus has been surgically repaired. She has a button for using a gastric tube that allows her to be fed through her stomach. She can't drink liquids, so that's a problem. She needs to be pump fed; she can't swallow well. She eats some food by mouth, actually only yogurt, blueberry yogurt. She's so opinionated and stubborn; she sure knows what she wants! She's a strong-willed child.

I'm thinking back on when I saw Kate for the first time in the ICU. My husband, Rich, was saying to the nurses, "You've got to tell the doctors to call her Kate, not baby. We gave her a name; make them use it." And I remember him fussing with her, handling a baby that is in really bad shape, playing with her, and saying, "It's okay, Katie," just like she was normal. He kept talking to her and giving her positive strokes. I know his heart was breaking. I think it was hurting him more than me. At that time, I couldn't get past my shock to even feel the hurt, yet Rich was reaching out and loving her. It was so beautiful. I was so moved.

A lot of beautiful things have happened between my husband and me since Kate was born. Very early on Rich and I made an unspoken pact that we wouldn't edit our feelings about Kate. Sometimes one of us will experience anger or disappointment, but we never keep our feelings from each other. I think it's good we aren't trying to protect each other or hide from our own feelings. This was and is important, a gift. It's one way we share this burden.

My husband and I had to eventually face what was true for us. We had to let go of trying to beat the predictions. It took a long time. These changes in how you think don't happen in an instant. We thought if we just tried harder, if we just asked more questions, if we just found out more, then we might find a cure, a solution, something, anything. For a time, we were consumed with thinking about what might be. Might she walk? Talk? And yet her critical clinical picture was often so severe that it overshadowed everything. The professionals wanted to keep trying with her, even though they didn't know for sure what her outcome would be. They didn't encourage us to institutionalize her, and frankly, I don't know what institution would have taken her.

I did what I needed to do, but it wasn't easy. For the first year of her life, my mothering instincts seemed to go away. I knew how to be a mom to my son, Richard, but with Kate I couldn't figure it out. I felt like a failure. I just didn't know how to be Kate's mom yet. I was like her case manager. I'd get involved with all kinds of specialists, doctors, and nurses. They would come to the house and suggest I try this or that, but every time I looked at her I couldn't get past the shock.

The turning point for me was when Kate got sick at the age of one year. She kept getting sicker and sicker, so we took her into the hospital, and she was there for over two weeks. It was a teaching hospital, and three waves of doctors saw her every day; they'd look at her like this specimen. I wanted them to see her as a child. I remember thinking that, even if she's a mess, she's so cute! I remember actually falling in love with her. I talked to the nurses about how great Kate was, and I'll bet they thought I was out of my mind. But I fell in love with her the way others had fallen in love with her before me. My mother just adored my child from the moment she was born. She picked out the beautiful stuff—her eyebrows, her fingers. She'd praise the good things. By the time we came home from that hospital stay with Kate, I finally felt like her mom. "Okay, this is it," I thought. "We aren't going to beat this. I'm going to be her mother. Other people can educate her and do her speech therapy. I'll mother her."

Most parents with kids like this keep thinking they'll find some new discovery, some new doctors with new information or some hopeful thing through a support group, but that gets old. No more fixing. I realized Kate would make small progress from time to time. My hopes and dreams for Kate to be normal had to go. I decided to look at what she gave me and be happy with whatever it was.

Kate is now ten years old. She's quite small. You might think she is only a couple of years old. She wears a size 5 dress. Kate doesn't talk, but she does communicate; she's quite clear about things. She's bright. I don't know what her IQ is, but I'd guess she's on the level of a two- or three-year-old. She knows where things she wants are in the house. If she wants something, like food, she will walk over, get me, and walk me to the refrigerator. She goes to a special school for multiply disabled children from nine to three, five days a week. She's in a very active program. It's like a preschool with smaller goals, but real goals. She's busy, and the ratio is three kids to one adult, so it's great.

Kate is so stimulated at the school during the week. Without those classes on the weekends she tends to get in trouble and she needs constant attention. When she's home, she requires structure. It's really hard. I just hired someone who will come and stay on Saturdays. That will give me a break. I need time away to do things, to take care of the other parts of my life.

Kate is actually fun to be with. My husband plays amazing games with her. He's kept his sense of humor and plays with Kate and laughs with her. It makes her more human to us, and that's healing. It's his way of really loving her and making her kid-like, not patient-like. Our son, Richard, for a while, didn't notice Kate much. Later on he became more aware of her. Then he'd ask when she was going to come to his school. I'd always say, "Well, she's taking her time," and I'd let him know she was slow. Now that Richard is twelve, he understands she won't ever catch up. He says some kids tease him about Kate. But the kids that come over to the house like her and actually play with her. Sometimes Richard scoops her up and sits her down with his friends. It's not perfect, but Kate is part of the family.

One day I had a discussion with a child psychiatrist at the hospital. I went into this whole thing about my worries and what might be in the future, and he said, "Stop! All we are really given is just this moment. That's it." Sometimes you're ready to hear what is being said, and I heard it. That conversation taught me something in a very deep way. The anxiety and worry shifted. What you can learn from having a child who could die at any minute is to live in the moment. It was a gift to me. Let's not worry about anything but whether she wakes up. And when she wakes up, we'll be present and in that moment. The future isn't part of my thinking.

To this day I still grieve the child I didn't have. I was very busy right after Kate was born, but when things were quiet I would have bouts of deep crying. I would see little kids who look a little like Kate and sink into depression. I remember a time when I took care of my niece for a day. I didn't think I could do it. I took her to the park, but by the end of the day I was sobbing. The contrast was too great.

Once I was in a panel discussion at Kate's school with other parents. The last question was "If you could have had anything from our community of support, what would you want?" I'm thinking things like a trip to a sunny place like the Bahamas or a housekeeper for a year—all sorts of things like that. A woman beside me spoke up and said, "You're basically asking me if you can take this away? No, you can't buy your way out. River runs through. There is no way out." I looked at her and realized she was so right. You don't get to take this away.

I want to have fun and have a normal life. We have parties and invite friends over. I want to be cheerful and happy. I have every reason to be depressed and angry, and I've been there.

Thank God, it fell away. I choose not to go there now. I am much less volatile, less anxious than I used to be. I've gotten over the feeling I had done something wrong to have this kid. I was healthy and I took good care of myself. This sad and unfortunate thing just happened. It is not my fault.

There are times now when, as the expression goes, I can actually "lighten up." I'm able to look back on situations in our household and smile, even laugh. Some circumstances are actually funny. When Kate was about five, my mother-in-law broke her hip and was confined to a wheelchair. She needed constant care and wasn't getting it at home. She lived with us for about a year and a half with twelve-hour-a-day professional care. Halfway through she had trouble swallowing. She finally got her own stomach tube and was fed like Kate. I remember one evening sitting at the table having dinner with my husband and our son. It was a normal dinner hour just like anybody else might have, except that Kate was buzzing around the living room and my mother-in-law was in the back room with a TV blaring while mumbling loudly to her aide. And that was our nutty household.

What are my hopes? I hope my husband and I will stay married. I know some relationships fall apart over these things. And I certainly hope our son will grow up healthy and become a good adult. I don't want him to suffer because of Kate. That's about it.

My husband and I probably will be caregivers for the rest of our lives. How we live is filtered through Kate's situation. It will be a life commitment for us. We need to start thinking about when we are too old to care for her anymore. But one thing we know for sure is that the most important thing for us is to have large wells of love for Kate and not let anything ever get in the way of that love we feel for her. She's the strangest mixture of bitter and sweet I've ever known and, for me, the dearest thing on earth.

Peg and her husband have learned a great deal about themselves as they've come to understand how to live comfortably with their daughter, Kate. It's easy to be sympathetic with such a situation but relatively impossible to imagine living and managing such a fragile and demanding situation. It's nearly impossible to know what new needs may unexpectedly arise, and to live with the awareness that each day can bring unexpected events and the necessity of quick decisions. I admire how Peg and her husband agreed to accept the responsibilities and possible challenges that may arise daily. They each demonstrate honest commitment to their daughter's needs with an attitude that makes their situation manageable and keeps their marriage solid.

1. **What are your thoughts and feelings about this story?**

2. **What stories do you know about other families with a child who was born needing special care—families that made different decisions about caring for their child? What decisions can you suggest that might offer a different result?**

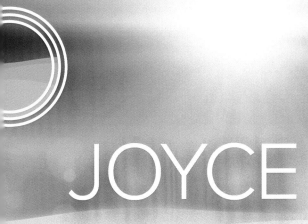

JOYCE

WHAT I WISH

WHEN I PHONED JOYCE, SHE INVITED ME TO COME TO HER HOME. I accepted her invitation and was delighted to spend the afternoon in her sunny living room, surrounded by memorabilia from exotic locations all over the world. Joyce told me that moving into this modest yet comfortable home was part of her adjustment to being an "I" after many years of being part of a "we." Two years earlier, Joyce's husband had died. Her work as a marriage and family therapist and a counselor for family caregivers provides many opportunities for her to reflect on her personal experience of caregiving. My encounter with her provided her with a chance to share her story.

My husband, Radcliff—I called him Rad—was a very healthy person. He ate right, exercised right, did everything right. Everyone went to Rad for health information; he was the authority on how to stay healthy. But there was one thing he didn't do when he had his annual physical exam, and that was to have the colonoscopy his doctor suggested. Knowing and dealing with the results of that test may have saved his life.

Soon after the diagnosis of colon cancer, Rad had a series of radiation treatments that were debilitating. After that, we took a vacation and pretended everything was normal. When we returned, we found the cancer had spread to his liver and one kidney. My caregiving experience began then; I rallied and became his full-time nurse. Rad was in and out of the hospital seven times in the following months. I wanted to help the person I loved, but it was hard. I was dealing adequately with the practical needs of the moment but not facing the possibility of my husband's death. Good friends would call and come over, and they'd say, "Do you want to talk about it?" I would say, "No, there's nothing to talk about," and I'd keep pretending it would all go away.

It never really occurred to me that my husband might die. I just kept thinking, "Well, we can see this through." I guess we thought that not thinking or talking about the death would keep it away. I never mentioned the possibility of his dying to Rad, and he never mentioned it to me. I just couldn't acknowledge that reality. After Rad died, I read an article about Lauren Bacall and Humphrey Bogart. Bogart was terribly sick with lung cancer, and it was obvious that he was never going to recover. "But we never said a word about it to each other," recalled Bacall. "It was like a secret, and if we didn't say it, then it wasn't going to be true." When I read that I thought, "Oh, sister, and I do mean *sister*!"

One day Rad went out to get the newspaper. When he came back in the house, he told me he couldn't focus his eyes. The doctor had warned me this would be a symptom that his kidneys had shut down. He never rallied after that. It was fourteen months from diagnosis to death. Rad was only sixty-four.

After Rad's death, I knew I needed help. I got a private trainer to come to my home and help my physically build myself up. I allowed myself to be with people, and I went out with my friends whenever they would ask. I let myself grieve. I believe you have to walk through the middle of the grief, because if you hide and try to avoid it, the grief will come on you later in some mental or physical problem. I've seen it happen many times. I don't minimize that I've had painful times and still do. But I think that I'm now a stronger person and much more compassionate toward others because I've seen my own weaknesses and failures.

The first month after Rad died, I didn't believe I could deal with all the details that needed attention. As I look back on our situation, I now feel strongly that unfinished business, financial matters and such, needs to be discussed openly and sensibly. Our denial of the reality of Rad's illness left me unprepared. In practical terms I was left in a mess financially, because we never talked about it. I think if Rad had seemed comfortable discussing finances, then I could have too. One of us needed to break through that wall of denial. Sadly, I've learned these things too late.

I'm learning now how to graciously accept help. I've always felt I should handle everything myself. I'm alone now, and I had to learn to accept help. I've been having some back problems, so I've even employed a gardener. One thing I understand now is that saying "No, no, no—I can do it myself" when people offer help actually shuts out the other person. They want to help, and insisting on being independent and taking care of everything yourself doesn't give them that opportunity.

My adult children tell me now that I never let them know how sick their father was. It was a terrible mistake. It kept our adult children separated from us and from the truth. I treated them like little children. Had Rad and I sat down with them and told them of their father's terminal illness, it could have been a far more meaningful experience for them. They would have come over and spent more time with us. If I had it to do over again, I'd be much more forthright about it all. I've learned to talk more openly about my feelings and fears with my children now, and that has helped me grow closer to them. Belated, that's true, but it has been a wonderful gift.

I can tell you another thing I've learned from my experience: caregivers need to take personal time off. I didn't do this, and it was a mistake that took a toll on me. Only a few times did I even let myself go for a walk, and once or twice I let myself go to lunch with a friend. I'd come back, and Rad would say, "You're a different person. I see in your face that you had a good time." That's what your loved one wants to see. They don't want to see you beaten down and haggard.

The thing that's most amazing is that for years I ran a caregivers' group and a widows' group at the center where I worked. It was my specialty. I was confident that I knew what there was to know about both of those areas. I had read a lot, talked to many people, was interviewed on a national radio broadcast on caregivers, and was well known for running successful caregiver groups. I guess I was a bit smug. But then I became a family caregiver and had to do all the things that people were always telling me about, like cleaning up vomit, changing soiled bed linen, and sitting hour after hour waiting for the doctor.

For all I thought I knew, I was also not prepared for the anger I felt. I hadn't really understood the anger caregivers talked about. As a counselor, I would say things like, "Your anger isn't helping; think how awful it is for your husband; blah, blah, blah." What did I really know? Now I had my own anger, and I'm sure my husband had his. I was also ashamed of being angry. I was mad at my whole situation. What had happened to my life, my plans? We were going to go to Italy; we had plans to go to Venice on our next vacation. We were financially secure, still young and vital. We had lots of years ahead of us. Our lives were good, and then everything changed.

Now when I counsel clients who are caregivers, I have a real understanding of their anger and where it's coming from, yet I sincerely believe that a person can grow from these hard experiences. I have seen people shut down, become very bitter, isolate themselves from the world, and let their anger become their overriding emotion. I was determined not to let that be the path for me. The enormous loss and grief I felt wasn't going to finish my life. I know my husband wouldn't have wanted that for me.

I've found that I'm now much more able to relate to the misfortunes of others—and in a deeper way. I'm able to bring a different level of sensitivity and feeling to the work I do. I find that I'm more emotionally available to my clients. I'm more tuned in to their feelings, I guess. Telling my story has made me a much more effective counselor.

Revealing your personal story is supposed to be a no-no for therapists, but in working with family caregivers, I've found it makes a real difference. My clients and I are able to relate on a whole different plane. I've been there. The thing I must always remember is that telling my personal story is for their benefit, not for mine.

It's been two years now since Rad died. I did the best I could, I guess, but I wish I had been able to deal with it more head-on. I've certainly experienced some profound personal growth, but of course I wish it all hadn't happened. It's hard when you've been part of a "we" to learn to be an "I" again. I'm not the person I was two years ago. I've grown, and I intend to keep growing. There still are lessons I can learn from this experience.

Upon reflection, Joyce sees that in both her personal caregiver experience and the way she and her husband handled his illness, in complete privacy, they were denying the reality of his illness even to themselves. She admitted that they were mistaken when they didn't share the truth of Rad's illness with their adult children. Neither of them acknowledged the possibility that Rad would require full-time care and that Joyce would become his caregiver. Their unrealistic attitude prevented them from making financial and legal arrangements and left Joyce with additional responsibility and stress after Rad's death. Of course, these practical matters aren't necessarily easy or comfortable to deal with. However, not being aware and informed was, she came to realize, poor judgment on their part.

1. When have you had an honest and open discussion with the person in care about the reality of his or her situation? What aspects of the diagnosis, prognosis, or treatment was the person in care able to accept and plan for?

2. Have you been in a situation where you were involved in a discussion about the diagnosis or treatment necessary for someone in the family? What were some of the reactions: denial, resistance, acceptance, support? How did the plan change as the person in care needed more assistance?

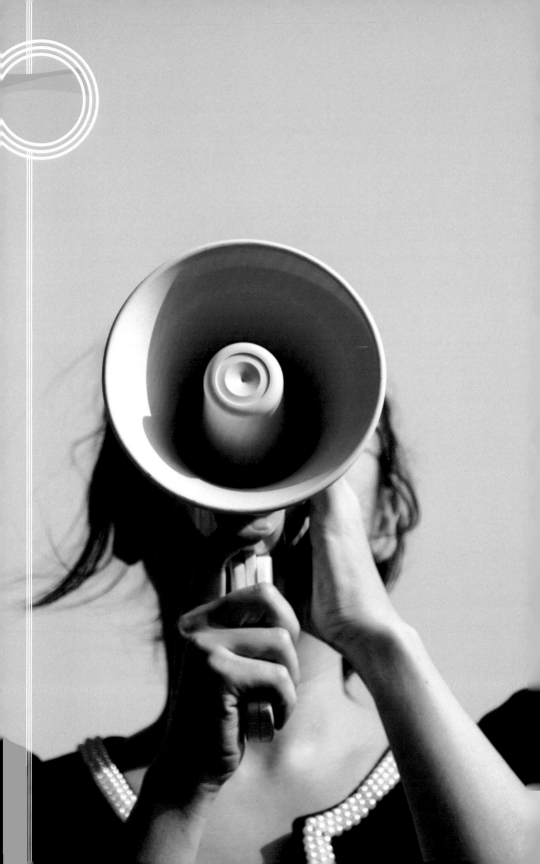

DANA

DANA IS THE WIFE AND PRIMARY CAREGIVER FOR HER HUSBAND, actor Christopher Reeve, who suffered a paralyzing spinal cord injury when he was thrown from his horse. Many of us remember him from his 1978 movie role as Superman. After you read this conversation with Dana, you might agree she deserves the label of Superwoman. I had an opportunity to meet and talk with her when I was producing a one-hour special for public radio, *Hardship into Hope: The Rewards of Caregiving.* Dana was most generous in discussing the changes and challenges and the profound learning that resulted from their situation. Our conversation took place a few years after her husband's accident. At the time, their son, Will, was six.

We now have a terrific relationship, but it took some doing. We didn't get married until five years after we met. Two of those years were a flurry of love and romance. The other years were knockdown, drag out— working out all the junk and making sure we both had equal footing and an agreed upon, real give-and-take. We knew marriage wouldn't always be pretty and perfect, and we talked about how we had to be there for each other. We hammered all that out, so by the time we got married, our eyes were wide open and we were more in love than ever. We really knew that we were choosing a partner for a lifetime—to go through the hard times and to survive the tough stuff with.

The accident instantly transformed life as our family knew it. Chris's life was changed. All our lives were changed, but his, of course, the most profoundly. He's the one that can't hop out of bed. He's the one that can't even scratch an itch. Those are huge changes.

I was able to cope better than I ever would have believed. Family rushed in; friends rushed in; neighbors were incredible. An energy came up for me; it was all about problem solving. Day by day, it was about getting things done—taking care of the insurance, filling out forms, talking with doctors—and I told myself, as many other women I've spoken with do, "I can do it, I can do it, I can do it. Whatever it is. I can do it, I can cope with it, and I can do it all." It takes a tremendous amount of energy, almost manic energy.

And then, about eighteen months into it, there is the settling and sinking realization and the slowing down—when you realize, okay, this is not a sprint. This is a long distance jog, and I'd better settle into a rhythm. Then along with that comes a down period for the caregiver and the recipient of the care too. For Chris and myself, and for the others in similar situations, there's that sobering realization that we not only have to endure what has already been endured, but we also have to continue to live like this. This is now the status quo. This is normal life.

One thing I've realized is that I'm part of a group called caregivers, and there are millions of us. Caregiving will someday touch all our lives. Former first lady Rosalynn Carter, in her book about caregiving, said something like, "You either have been a caregiver, you are going to be caring for someone, or you're going to need to be cared for." It's often something that we take on willingly, because we love the person or because we feel it's our duty. And yet we don't see it as a job, necessarily, and it really is. Not that we wouldn't do it anyway.

I do realize that I'm in a position that many, many other people are not—a situation of privilege. I'm able to have people help me out with things like housework. I'm able to have a babysitter. And I don't have to worry about how much that costs. We have other financial resources we can count on. So that removes a tremendous amount of stress that I just don't have to experience. Yet, I realize that many, many people live with that stress.

For the first ten months I was doing most of the physical care myself and training the staff we have now. I slowly weaned myself from the physical care. My caregiving now is almost entirely emotional. The more difficult task, I find, is that emotional caregiving. I remember once reading an article, before Chris's injury, about a woman whose husband suffered chronic depression over a long period of time and about how difficult it was for her to be his caregiver. I remember I thought that surely she could get away from that or handle it some way, and I passed it off. I think of that now and realize how smug my response was.

I know now that in many ways, dealing with a loved one's depression and negative emotions is more difficult than the physical care. I can lift all day long. I can wipe a face or wipe a bottom. There's a beginning, a middle, and an end to those tasks. You do it, you've achieved it, and it's done. Dealing with someone's emotions is much more complicated, much messier, much more ongoing. I've grown a lot in my understanding. I'm not so sure how to really describe it all. But the reality of the hardship of everyday life is much more present. Our life is about compromise and coping with difficulties. I'm doing a good deal of that, and I think I've really grown.

I have never really plunged into despair. I have down moments, but I can honestly say they're not very frequent. Something that Chris often speaks about is that when he feels the most down and the sorriest for himself, he focuses on other people and what he can offer them. That helps him out of his funk. Chris talks with and helps a lot of young kids who've had spinal cord injuries. A lot of people who have spinal cord injuries, especially young men in their late teens and early twenties, talk with him about wanting to die. He knows how to deal with them and helps them understand that compromise is going to be a way of life; that it feels lousy now, but you're going to be okay and handle it. Chris has talked to a couple of kids and truly has saved their lives. He's been incredible that way. And what he does bolsters him.

And I find the same thing for myself when I speak to groups (particularly to women who are caregivers) about strategies to survive difficulty. I find that it reenergizes me. I feel like I'm doing something worthy. I'm producing good out of bad. Chris and I have helped a tremendous number of people. I speak on the subject of nurturing the nurturer and how important it is for caregivers to do good things for themselves. Caregivers need to give themselves permission to do something self-indulgent, relaxing, and completely removed from their caregiver responsibilities. You need to find ways to sustain yourself for the long haul. The person needing care always has needs to be filled, whether they're emotional or physical, so caregivers must take time for themselves.

What Chris is able to give back to me is the same thing he's able to give to the world. He inspires me. There's something about being with somebody with a disability who, against all odds, achieves the goals he sets for himself that can't help but be inspiring to those around him. You really don't feel like you can complain about your own problems, and, truly, you don't even feel like complaining when you see someone who is dealing with a life that's so difficult moment to moment and not only getting through it but also doing so much for others.

I so admire how he handles his job as a parent, as a father. His job is doubly hard. Chris would love to be able to be out there coaching some of the sports that Will plays. But he goes to the games if the weather isn't too cold and cheers our son on. Chris loves hockey—he played it in high school and college—and would have loved to be out there with him. Now he puts his feelings aside, and it hurts him, I know. He makes the effort to go to the games to support Will.

I'm always aware of how much joy I get out of physical activity, of being able to take Will places easily, to hop on a subway in New York and go to a museum. When we plan something as a family, there's the whole logistical thing: going in back entrances, making special arrangements, things like that. I'm so aware and appreciative of how easy things are for me. If I were in bed and couldn't get up and couldn't go outside, I think it would really depress me. I know that's what Chris goes through.

Chris is very conscious of remaining a vibrant, vital part of the family. He's a giving husband and a partner. We place the same demands on one another that we've always asked of each other. We have to live up to the other's expectations every day. It's how we live.

I never would have asked for something like this to happen. And yet, the fact is that it didn't stop our life. It changed the direction of our life. I'm surprised in retrospect by how much joy we still have. I think if someone had presented this scenario to me, had said my husband would be in a sudden, debilitating accident, I would not have felt I would be able to cope with the situation at all or that our life would still have any happiness. I think that's what a lot of people imagine. It actually turned out to be quite the contrary.

Real gifts come along with the hardship, and, if not for Chris's accident, I'm not sure we would have ever known these. We have a tremendous amount of joy in our family, a tremendous amount of laughter. We're a very close family. For example, one small thing: Chris isn't well today, so he has to stay in bed. This means we'll all have dinner together in the bedroom. We'll sit in a circle around the bed, because we want to have our meal together. We'll have a pleasant dinner hour together. It will make Chris feel good, and it keeps us living and sharing as a family. It sends a powerful message that no matter what your physical condition, you are a valued member of the family, and we're going to carry on in our way together.

We're all so grateful for a beautiful day, so grateful for sunshine, for a day when Chris can be outside and not feel cold. I don't mean to sound like everyone isn't thankful for a beautiful day, but there is something about the fact that we've learned to truly appreciate the simple things, and I know I can experience joy and happiness even during difficult times. That's certainly one very powerful insight, and I don't think anyone could have told me that this was true. I've learned that you must live your life fully and well and try to appreciate what you've got.

This change in our lives has affected our son, Will. He's become incredibly caring about other people. He's very physically affectionate, very concerned that other people's feelings and needs are taken care of, and he's wonderfully giving. He's also very accepting of people regardless of what they look like, what they can or cannot do. I think all this is a result of living with a father who has a disability. I make a conscious effort not to present to Will the world as a fearful and dangerous place. And yet the other side of that is that anything can happen. Accidents can happen to anyone.

Both Chris and I have learned something about parenting from our situation. So much of parenting is being there for the child. It's not so much being able to throw a ball, for example, as sharing the child's experience, being there to support the child in throwing the ball. And then there's the big lesson. One of the greatest tools we can give our children is the capacity to deal with hardship and still have a happy life. We've been given this gift just by virtue of the fact that this accident happened. Life is going to be painful at times; we're all going to have our pain, loss, frustration, and hardship. The best things we can give our children are the tools to cope. You can adapt, you can find ways to be happy, and these are tremendously valuable lessons.

Whether we like it or not, we've become role models. And that's both a burden and a gift. If we perceive it more as a gift and less as a burden, it feels better. We've been given a caregiver's soapbox. The system has not recognized the reality of family caregivers. By family caregiver, I mean a person responsible for the care of a spouse, parent, child, or other family member who is disabled or ill. That responsibility isn't officially recognized, not even on the census form. We need to start changing the system to provide some kind of financial aid for the job of family caregiving. The amount of money that family caregivers are saving the health-care system by taking on this responsibility is enormous. What a wonderful thing it would be if we could, as a society, acknowledge these values of wanting to keep the care of family members in the family, wanting to take care of our own. I really feel gratified that by speaking out, Chris and I are able to make a difference, and that's another fight we've taken on as a result of our situation.

New awareness and necessary learnings came into Dana's life as she settled into her role of caregiving for her husband, Chris. Her new commitment began unexpectedly with Chris's serious injury and, like many, began with Dana taking on everything that was needed in this new and demanding situation. Many family members have told me that at first they take over everything needed in their particular caregiver situation. Their mantra is similar to Dana's words: "I can do it. I can do it. I can do it. I can do it all!" Many caregivers soon experience exhaustion and depression, and often become ill. A solo commitment isn't the wisest solution for those taking on these new responsibilities. Wise caregivers talk with others in the family and figure out who else can help with some chore or responsibility in this new and demanding situation. As I so often say to family caregivers, "Take care of yourself, so you can take care of another."

Dana talked about her son, Will, and the importance of facing the reality of his father's situation while continuing to be included in his daily life. Some parents feel a need to protect or shield younger children from an illness or arrange for them to spend only limited time with the person now requiring care. I don't support that idea. Honest and open sharing at their level of understanding, I believe, is necessary for children.

This book has been updated and reprinted, and visibility for family caregivers is now openly discussed and covered in the press, compared to the situation at the time of my interview with Dana. Support groups, opportunities for respite events, and many church and community assistance programs have been activated and are eagerly attended and supported. Persons who have served as a family caregiver are often left exhausted and separated from their work and social life when their caregiving responsibility comes to an end. A new trend, although still in a beginning stage in limited locations, are support groups for these recovering caregivers, who often aren't ready to immediately return to work and the social world of an active and busy society.

Families often spend a good deal of their income and savings on medications, relief help, and payment for other services. One issue that is often discussed but still unsupported is a plan for making funding available to lower middle-class and low income families to supplement the care needed. I hope that in the future, the full-time job a family caregiver takes on will be acknowledged by legislation that provides either hourly pay or some financial compensation for the primary family caregiver.

1. **What stories can you share of keeping children involved in the daily life of a parent who requires caregiving?**

2. **How are meals managed in your particular situation? Is the person in care part of family meals? Why or why not? How could meals be shared, at least on certain days or in some specific situations? What would sharing meals mean for the person in care?**

NORTON AND BEV

THE LEGACY THEY LEFT US

THESE DAYS WE HEAR A LOT ABOUT MIDDLE-AGED CHILDREN taking care of aging parents. As life spans lengthen, increasing numbers of "children" now into their sixties and seventies are taking care of elderly parents. This was the situation for Norton and Bev, a brother and a sister, both in their sixties. The day their dad stumbled on the steps, knocking over their mother as he fell and causing her to break her hip, Norton and Bev decided it would be best for their parents to come and live with them. They told me of their deep love, respect, and admiration for their parents, who, Norton said, had left them "a legacy on how to make the world a better place in which to live."

I was invited to come to Norton and Bev's home to talk with them about their caregiving experience. The dining room table was covered with photos of their parents and other mementos. It was obvious that this had been a close and caring relationship. Norton began our conversation.

Our folks lived with us for almost five years. It was probably an advantage that neither of us is married. We didn't have the other family concerns and obligations that many people have, so we were able to devote full attention to taking care of our parents.

During those years when my sister and I were caregiving, we were together as a family all the time. Through good times and bad, we got very close. Our mother was fragile in her last years and could barely talk. She was very weak, yet how she handled her diminished health taught us something important. She was a caring, gentle, and considerate person, always thanked people who were helping her, and was able to smile, right up to the end.

I used to travel a lot, but during those years when Mother and Dad lived with us, I gave that up. I knew someday my role as a caregiver would end, and I'd do my traveling then. Mother died when she was ninety. About ten days before she died, she told me how much she appreciated that we had taken care of her and thanked us for all we had done for her. It was amazing that she could summon up the energy to say that. It meant a lot to both my sister and me.

Dad always had an upbeat attitude. About three or four days before he passed away, I remember saying to him, "Hey, you seem to feel a little better today," and he smiled and said, "Why not?" He never made a big thing about small stuff. His attitude was always positive, and you could hear it in his favorite phrase, "Why not?"

Bev came into the room at that point, talking about her father as she served us tea.

Just thinking of Dad now as we talk warms my heart, because he was so full of energy for life and laughter, and he enjoyed everything so much. Everyone in his presence felt this sense of joy too. There was always a warm conversation, and I always seemed to be learning new things from him. He continued to teach me how to be a good person and also how to be religious and observe religious holidays with meaning. He taught us to enjoy life and make the most of each day. Both Mother and Father were strong in their beliefs. Mother had her concerns about social equality, and Dad had his religious convictions and practices. Their example taught us to stand up for what we believe.

In his later years, Dad did have some dementia, but we continued to have conversations and enjoy each other's company. It helped to keep my dad alert. I kept talking to him all the time, even when we were watching television. I'd say things like, "That man on TV has a red tie just like yours" or "Oh, look at that person's blue eyes." It would keep his mind active. He worked hard to remember things and keep thinking, because he knew he had some memory lapses and confusion. He never really lost touch. He knew both of us by name until the end. We always took him places with us.

My brother and I didn't want him to think of himself as being different and unable to function in a social situation. Sometimes he would drop things on the floor or make a mess at the table, but we weren't embarrassed. We would clean it up, continue the dinner conversation, and we were glad to have him with us. He always liked to feel important, so we kept our attention on him when we were with others. If he had been in a nursing home, he probably would have just been sitting there, but we kept him doing things as long as he could. At the end he lost his mobility and had difficulty standing up, so we had some help come into the house, because we realized that *we* needed some help. But up until then my brother and I managed the care he needed.

I know that Norton and I never regretted what we gave up to take care of our mother and father. We had good times with them up until the end, and we were blessed because we had friends and family around. People were always in the house. Everything we did for our parents was with love. The legacy they left us is love.

I haven't often heard of family caregiving living arrangements coming together as easily as they did for Bev and Norton. That the sister and brother were both single and sharing a home made their caregiver obligations more manageable. In many ways, this family situation was unique in these times when adult children often live great distances from their parents. When the care of a parent becomes necessary and family help is required, often either the parents or one of their adult children moves, causing drastic changes in the daily life of the one who moves. Bev and Norton's situation was easily and comfortably resolved, because everyone was living in the same city.

The relationship of Bev and Norton with each of their parents wasn't characterized by inconvenience and hardship; it was one of respect, love, and sincere dedication to giving care to each parent in need. They never thought twice about providing the care each required, and both Bev and Norton moved relatively easily into their caregiver roles. Living in the same city, and eventually having their parents move into their home, made caring for their parents convenient and comfortable for Bev and Norton.

1. Do you know of situations in which a parent or both parents moved in with one of their children to be cared for? Has the situation been agreeable and comfortable, or have plans needed to be altered? If new arrangements had to be made, how and for what reasons were they changed?

2. In Bev and Norton's telling of their story, they emphasized the element of love. Was it a surprise to you? As many caregivers certainly care deeply about their parents, what might be some reasons that love for a parent is so rarely mentioned?

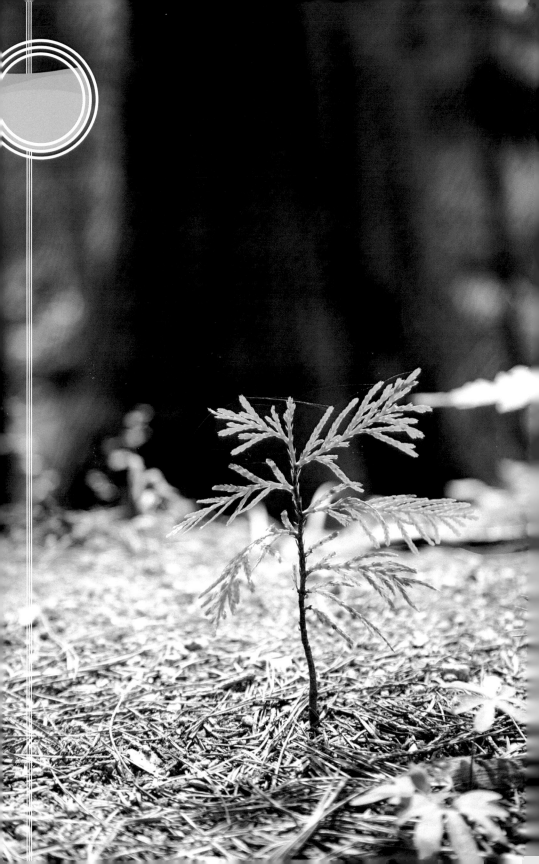

RACHAEL

I'VE REALLY GROWN UP

WHEN I MET RACHAEL, SHE WAS THE TEENAGE KID OF MY LAND-
lord, Richard, a creative and brilliant architect. I had taken a job
far from my hometown and needed to lease a small apartment.
I moved into the third floor of a charming building that housed
Richard's office and the offices of two other architects. We became friends, the kind of friends you make an effort to hold on
to when you move. Many years later, Rachael and I were both living in the Los Angeles area when I heard about Richard's stroke
and that her father would be relocating to an apartment near her.
That's how we all ended up once again living in the same city, and
that's how Rachael and her dad became a chapter in this book.

I don't really think of myself as a caregiver. When I think of
a caregiver, I think of someone who is more involved with
daily care. My dad isn't that dependent and he isn't bedridden. He gets around, makes some of his own meals, brushes
his teeth, and bathes himself. He can go to the store, count
change, things like that. At this time, he doesn't require high
maintenance like many caregiver stories you probably hear.

Yet, I guess I'm in this for the long haul, so in that sense you could call me a caregiver. When my dad was fifty-eight, he had a stroke. That was about twelve years ago, and it left him unable to speak or write.

It was a real tragedy, because he was a creative and successful architect. Now his only method of communication is drawing pictures and pantomiming. I'm his main link with the outside world. My communication with him is basically a game of twenty questions. As he gets tired, later in the evening, it gets more difficult for him to communicate, and the harder he tries, the harder it is for him to get the words out, so it can become frustrating. We live a couple of blocks from each other, and not a day goes by without my stopping over to bring something, pay his bills, watch over his portfolio, or deal with other things related to his care. I've had to take on all this and learn about it. That learning curve for me was difficult; it requires continual rearranging of my life.

My parents were living on the East Coast when Dad had the stroke. My mom took charge of everything; I had already moved away from home. Then my mom died quite unexpectedly. That was five years ago, and that's when I came into the picture. Dad moved to the city where I live. My only sister had died quite young, so I was the only immediate family he had left. For a period of time, after my mother died, things got really difficult for me. It was just too much. I had to pack up their whole house and move everything into a place near me. Moving Dad to a strange city eliminated many of his activities and took away the few friends he had. The move was very stressful for both of us.

I guess what happened then was that I got caught up in the minutiae of things and lost track of the big picture. I had taken a three-month leave of absence from my work, and we were spending a lot of time playing cards together. Meanwhile, I hadn't done any interviews to find caregivers for when I went back to work. I hadn't gone out to check on different living situations for him, and I hadn't made any effort to replace some of the activities and services he had before he moved here. I sort of became a little girl and lost my confidence to go out in the world and make adult, responsible decisions. I was hiding behind games of gin rummy.

But, you know, my mother had just died, my dad had unexpectedly become my responsibility, and I was angry and depressed; now I realize my dad was too. I think most of my anger was really aimed at my mother. When she unexpectedly died I felt she had abandoned both of us. I hadn't had any time to work out the loss of my mom. I didn't know what to do with my feelings. I ended up feeling very guilty, because I would dump on my dad, and that sure wasn't fair. I finally realized I needed therapy and medication. I needed to get my own life on track again.

I've now learned to ask for help when I need it. That's my big learning out of this experience. I believed that if you wanted something done, you had to do it yourself. I've now learned that in your caregiving responsibilities you can't do everything yourself. A caregiver can't survive that way. We need other people—friends, contacts, neighbors, and professional help too. I've learned to reach out to others.

My mother never could do this. She was a 24/7 caregiver, and she took care of Dad all the time, never asking anyone for help, never living her own life. Toward the end of her life, when she was dying of lung cancer, a friend of the family came over to visit. She noticed that my mom could barely get out of bed and told my dad that something wasn't right. As well as he could, my dad said to this lady, "Yes, yes, she's sick," but my mom just wouldn't give in and ask for help. I lived in another city, and my mom didn't tell me how things were with her. When she finally got medical help, we discovered that my mom's lung had collapsed. She died one week later. She had no medical care prior to that. I think Mom was stubborn and in denial because she didn't know what would happen to Dad if she wasn't there to care for him.

Like my mom, I didn't understand how to reach out to others or that they'd be there for me if I asked for help. Yet I really needed to rely on others. Now I've arranged for friends and neighbors to take Dad places when I'm at work. I've learned to ask others to drive him to appointments, bring him to his stroke support group, go with him to the market or his speech therapy class, and take him to his tai chi class. Asking others for help has made possible those things that make his life better.

Some of my friends have asked why I didn't just have my dad move in with me, instead of going to all the trouble and expense of setting him up in his own place. Well, first of all, the independence is better for him. But the other thing is that I've had a pattern of merging too easily into my parents' lives, and these past five years or so I've been working hard to establish my own life and separate what my needs and wants are and to really become my own person. I had to avoid a situation where I was just my dad's caregiver and daughter. If this had all happened ten years earlier, that's what would have happened; I would have dropped everything in my own life. I've grown a lot since then, but I look back and know that I probably would have quit my job, stayed at home, been the good daughter, always there at his side. That's what my mom did, and I would have just taken over her role.

I've come to grips with the fact that it isn't within my ability to make Dad happy. I know he's somewhat depressed; he's had his share of losses. But I can only do what I can do, and I've accepted that reality. The other thing I've learned is that I have a lot of patience, and knowing that has certainly helped. My friends will witness Dad trying to communicate something to me, how long it takes, and it makes them nervous. I just sit and wait, as I've learned that it takes persistence and patience, and thankfully I've discovered I've got both. I've learned a lot about myself through a new understanding of my dad's problems. I've really grown up. I never would have believed in my wildest dreams that I was actually capable of doing all this stuff. Being able to handle all these family challenges has built up my self-confidence.

My partner and I often discuss our retirement, and we talk about having a house with an attached apartment for Dad. He's part of our long-term picture and our plans. Dad is seventy now and in almost perfect physical health. One day I was joking with him and I said, "You know, in thirty years when you're one hundred and in a wheelchair, I'll probably be in one too." For a moment we laughed at the idea of us both going down the street in wheelchairs. Then we both started to cry, because it could actually happen.

Rachael's story is about more than her accepting the responsibility of the family caregiver. It's about her personal growth. Although still in her twenties, Rachael's continued responsibility for her father gave her the gift of maturity.

What can we learn as we read this caregiver story? It seems that her parents were very private people, never sharing any details of their lives with whatever family they had, or with friends and neighbors. It wasn't a surprise that Rachael took on all the family needs alone. Possibly because of her young age, she wasn't aware of the local agencies and religious organizations that exist specifically to offer help and suggestions for family care-givers, and she didn't think to share her situation with neighbors or friends of the family. Assuming a family caregiving responsi-bility in such a seemingly secret and private way isn't always the wisest or most useful decision.

1. What stories do you know about situations where a care-giver could benefit from neighbors' help or assistance but the caregiver doesn't ask? Without feeling like an intruder, how might a neighbor be of help in some way?

2. How might neighbors or friends offer help when the person who has taken on the responsibilities of a family caregiver is overly protective of privacy?

3. What other questions come to mind about this very private and individual approach to caregiver responsibilities?

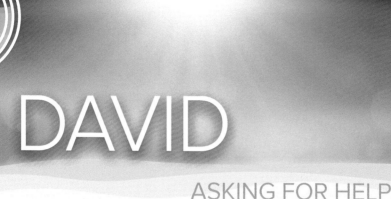

DAVID

ASKING FOR HELP

WHEN I VISITED DAVID IN HIS NEW YORK CONDOMINIUM, IT had been three months since his partner, John, had died of complications from AIDS. They had been together seven years; David's first partner had died more than ten years earlier. At the time John met David, John worked in the music industry for ASCAP, the American Society of Composers, Authors and Publishers. It's a field he enjoys, because music is a big part of his life. When I talked with David, John's death was so recent that he was barely back in his normal work routine. "I'm realizing that it takes time to heal," David told me. He talked about how he had grown from his caregiving experiences, but he also shared that it had been "hard-earned wisdom." In a choked voice and with sadness in his eyes, David said, "I want to tell you my story, our story." And so he began.

We were both HIV positive when we met. In the seven years I had known John, he was sick on and off, but he'd bounced back from serious bouts before. We both naïvely believed he'd come through the recent setback, but this time he really didn't. Gradually over the last six months of his life John lost a great deal of weight, couldn't eat solid foods, and couldn't swallow. When he came home from the hospital for the last time, he needed a suction machine, tube feedings, and the help of a home care worker. The last couple of months I slept on the sofa bed, because John's hours were erratic and the machines were so noisy. As the cancer metastasized, he developed pneumonia and went into cardiac arrest. John died just three months ago.

As sick as John was, I must admit that we never looked at the situation realistically. He had rebounded so many times in the past, even from a stroke three years ago, that we never anticipated he might not recover. I guess I expected that because so many medical advances had come about in recent years, there would be something new to pull him through. I realize now that neither of us was willing to see the reality. It was terrible for me when I came to realize that neither medical help nor anything I could do would save him.

Because we both were avoiding reality, we didn't take care of the practical things we should have at that time. We didn't prepare realistically. John's estate is now going into probate; our condo is going to have to be sold, and I'm left with all this on top of the loss and grief I deal with every day. This is a very hard time for me. Maybe for some of us it's our human nature to hide in denial. Anyhow, that's how we coped.

The last day John was here at home, he asked me to lie down beside him. I'm crying now when I look back on that day. I think he realized he was close to dying and wouldn't be coming back home from his next trip to the hospital. These were our last moments of intimacy. Even at the end, the love between us was as strong as it had ever been. When they took John off life support, he kept breathing on his own for most of the week. Some of his family and friends kept a vigil night and day. At some point, I could see I needed some time off, and I went home and was alone for the first time in days. I sat there and realized I couldn't go on holding my breath. I had been in suspended animation, on the edge, in a daze, and in a twilight zone for days. Then, for the first time, I started to feel that John could finally relax and let go.

Now I'm doing what I have to do to make things easier for myself. I write in my journal about the pain I'm feeling when I'm in the depths of my grief and depression. It helps to get it out on the page. I'm now in an online cancer-caregivers support group, and through it I've become friendly with a man whose wife of fifty years had cancer and another man who's the primary caregiver for his mother. My connection with these men, although I have actually never met them, has been enormously supportive. My parents live in Florida, and I haven't seen them since John's death, but they call often, and they too have been very supportive.

Now people have been reaching out to me here in my community, and that's a gratifying thing. I've had some dinner invitations, and the woman next door had two of her friends come over one day to clean my apartment. The people I work with raised some money in the office to help pay some of the funeral expenses, and others in the neighborhood often inquire how I'm doing. I never realized what being part of a community could offer.

When friends or neighbors ask what they can do for me, it seems to work best if I suggest something specific. I sometimes tell them that I'd like it a lot if they'd come and visit on Tuesday or Wednesday, or I specifically suggest that we could go to dinner together and share an evening. I'm finding that it still remains rather hard for me to initiate a call to ask someone to do something for me. During the first couple of weeks after John's death, there were a lot of messages on the phone machine and cards in the mail, but then that dropped off. I'm learning that it's my job now to continue to reach out to others. That's my part of the responsibility to keep connected. I've come to understand that it's a survival technique that has rewards.

When you have a committed, loving relationship and expect to spend the remainder of your life with that person, and death ends that, the loss is heavy and the grief is deep. Now that I'm alone, like so many others in similar situations, I have to learn how to nurture myself. I need to give myself the credit, love, and support I've been giving to others. It's my nature to give, and I've been privileged to do that with two partners. In a sense, I gave each of my partners at the time the best years of their lives. I've grown both from caregiving experiences and from the grief and loss I've endured. Yet it's been hard-earned wisdom. I trust there will be good things in my life ahead, so I hold on. I hope I will love again. I have a lot of love to share.

Some readers might think that David's story is in this book because our society has grown more aware of same-sex couples. Although that's an important change over the past few decades, the primary reason for sharing David's story is that, like David, many families cannot face the gravity of their situation, perhaps that there may not be a cure for the person in care. Both David and John were not able or willing to deal with the practical side of this very emotional situation. The result for them, and regrettably the result in many other situations, was financial and property loss along with the grief of John's death.

David also talked about his time of grief and the welcome attention from neighbors and friends. I believe his method of responding to offers for help by asking for specific things, time together, or other help is important for us to hear about. I've learned of many situations where pride or the desire to show one's strength and ability to handle the death of a loved one gets in the way of accepting help. Asking outright for help is even more difficult for many.

David's way of negotiating with those who are offering help works well for him and seems sensible in general. Only the grieving person knows whether he needs someone to pick up groceries, to join him for a dinner or movie evening out, to pick him up for a neighborhood event or a doctor appointment. We need to accept that others' offer to help is sincere, and we each need to tell people what they can do to help.

1. Have you been in a situation where immediate family members are unable or unwilling to accept the impending death of the person in care? What have you learned from such an experience? Have you been able to help others in such circumstances? How can you as a professional, a neighbor, or a friend help someone face an impending death and deal sensibly with practical matters while offering emotional support too?

2. Have you had experiences related to grief and loss with

same-sex couples? What stories can you share related to the reactions and responses from neighbors? Have these been positive or negative? How have you responded to such experiences?

3. Many people are no longer avoiding speaking about death. What do you think and feel about this type or discussion, and why?

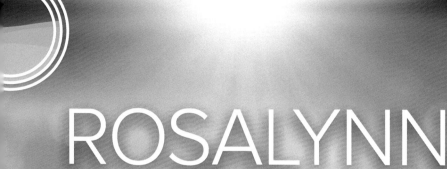

ROSALYNN

FOUR KINDS OF PEOPLE

IN 1999 I PRODUCED AN HOUR-LONG PUBLIC RADIO PROGRAM entitled *Hardship into Hope: The Rewards of Caregiving.* This book grew out of the positive response to the broadcast. One voice in that radio program was of former first lady Rosalynn Carter, wife of former president Jimmy Carter. I was fortunate to be able to arrange a conversation with Mrs. Carter, who wrote about the concerns of family caregivers in her book *Helping Yourself Help Others,* published in 1994. Here are some of Rosalynn Carter's comments from our meeting.

An enormous number of us at some time in our lives will take on the responsibility of caring for another person who is ill or incapacitated, or we ourselves will possibly be the one in need of care. Caregiving has certainly touched my life and my family. My father died when I was thirteen, the oldest of four children. My mother depended heavily on me to help her. Her mother, my grandmother, died the next year, and my grandfather came to live with us. He was seventy at the time, and he lived to be ninety-five. When my mother also needed care in her later years, I was traveling so much that I couldn't give her the full-time care she required. When she was ninety-two, we made the very difficult decision to move her into an assisted living facility. It was a decision that was painful for us, as it is for many families, but she couldn't stay by herself any longer.

My daughter-in-law was thrust into the role of family caregiver when her father died. Her mother, who lived five hours away, was miserable living by herself. She was equally miserable when she came to visit her daughter. It was a very stressful situation. At the time they had three little boys, so my daughter-in-law had to take care of her mother and the children, a common situation in many families. So, I've experienced a whole range of caregiving in my family. I've also worked a good deal with people who were caring for the mentally ill. Ever since my husband was governor of Georgia in the early 1970s, the whole issue of caregivers has been very important to me.

When we came to Atlanta from the White House, our local college had a small endowment for mental health programs.

We began working with persons who cared for the mentally ill. Our first big session focused on the issue of caregiver burnout. It also was open to people who were caring for those who were physically handicapped, frail, or elderly. This modest program started us working with caregivers in our community. When we established the Rosalynn Carter Institute, no other group we knew of was working on the issue of caregiving. I called more than thirty organizations, and not one had a program on caregiving. These days people realize that family caregivers need support systems for themselves and for those in their care.

People might be surprised to learn that family members or friends attend to most persons needing care at home. Only 10 to 20 percent of those requiring care receive it from professional caregivers. Employers are recognizing the need to create support programs for their employees who, more and more, are regularly checking on loved ones at home, taking them to appointments, and attending to their many needs. These caregivers need support systems at the workplace as they juggle home and work responsibilities.

When we first began our program, we interviewed hundreds of family caregivers. Almost every caregiver we talked with felt guilty if they weren't always with their loved one or on call every minute of every day. Many felt overwhelmed, isolated, and overly burdened. But if a person can develop the attitude that caregiving is a volunteer job they've taken on, and something they've entered into willingly to help a loved one, they feel freer to ask for outside help. In some situations they hire help either part time or full time, depending on what's needed and what a family can afford.

Caregiving is very difficult. I always say that if you don't take care of yourself, then the quality of care you give to your loved one is diminished. The message I would like to give to all caregivers, no matter what their personal situation, is that they must find some space in the day just for themselves. Make time, make space, have something outside your caregiving that's your own. Get out if you can. Some caregivers can't, but they can have hobbies or other activities that relax and distract them and give them pleasure. One woman, who was responsible for caring full time for her mother and tending her mother's large garden too, recently told me she started taking photographs of the flowers. She ended up setting up a business selling her photographs!

When we did our survey, even the people whom we felt were the most burdened would tell us that they found much satisfaction and many rewards in caregiving. I remember talking with one woman who said, "I just wanted to run away from it all, and one day I did. I checked into a motel, left my father all alone in a wheelchair, stayed there a couple of hours before I felt so guilty that I went home." And then she said, "I can take better care, more loving care, of my father than anybody!" She felt real pride that she could do that, that she could do something to make someone else's life better.

It's important and extremely satisfying to keep communications open with the ones you're caring for. Let them share their feelings and fears with you too. You can say something like, "I know how you must feel about this happening to your body. You must be sad; you must be angry." Acknowledging their feelings and fears makes communication so much easier. They can see then that you have compassion and empathy for them.

Physical touch is also really important. People who are ill feel helpless, damaged; that they're a burden. They no longer feel physically attractive or that they're lovable. For someone to touch them, put a hand on their brow or hold their hand, can make them feel that somebody really cares for them no matter how they look or feel or what is wrong with them. You must let yourself feel the sadness, the frustration, the pain, and the anger of your loved one. And you must grieve your loved one's losses and your own.

If the media told good stories of family caregivers coping with their many challenges, stories about the trauma and stress of having to put a loved one in a home or other facility, and the sadness one experiences in giving up their own home, it would let caregivers know that they're not alone, that these things touch everyone. Caregivers often feel they're isolated, that nobody cares about them, that what they're doing is thankless. It's important to let people know that caregiving for somebody is a very important thing, a very meaningful thing for a person to be able to do.

Profound learning often comes with caregiving. Hearing stories of caregivers helps prepare us all to be caregivers someday. Every household is going to face this issue at one time or another in some way. Like I've said before, there are only four kinds of people in this world: those who have been caregivers, those who currently are caregivers, those who will be caregivers, and those who will need caregivers. That pretty much covers all of us.

This now updated edition of the book gives me the opportunity to thank Rosalynn Carter for her wisdom and insight about the enormous growth in family caregiving, which has occurred as this country's oldest generations live longer and require care into their eighties, nineties, and even hundreds. Indeed, the number of family caregivers in the United States is now somewhere around 65 million. Fortunately, the term *family caregiver* is now in most Americans' vocabulary. Unfortunately, financial aid is not available from our national or state governments for either partial or full-time caregiving for a family member.

However, there is a growing awareness of the truth of Rosalynn Carter's words. "There are only four kinds of people in this world: those who have been caregivers, those who currently are caregivers, those who will be caregivers, and those who will need caregivers. That pretty much covers all of us."

1. Share either your personal caregiver story or another experience or encounter with a family caregiver that came to mind when you read Rosalynn Carter's comments. What thoughts or learning has this story raised for you?

2. What changes related to family caregiving are you aware of in laws, support groups, or services now available through churches and other groups, whether for free or for a charge?

3. How has family caregiving become visible in your community or in other locations in the United States?

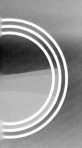

ARDITH

IT TAKES A FAMILY

IN MY TRAVELS I'VE MET MANY PEOPLE WHO COULD BE CONSID-
ered long-distance caregivers—daughters, sons, grandchildren,
nieces, cousins, in-laws, relatives of all varieties who manage to
participate in some way in a loved one's care from a distance.
That responsibility often necessitates extensive travel, sometimes
a weekend trip, often an extended stretch of time, whatever it
takes to supervise and coordinate care. Each situation is managed differently, and every circumstance requires unique compromises. "You do what you feel you must do," Ardith told me
when we talked about her caregiving responsibilities for her
mother and father. I arrived for my scheduled appointment with
her on a Friday afternoon, and her car was packed for her regular

weekend trip to see her parents. When we finished our conversation, she drove away before I even got into my car. She had a much longer drive to her destination than I did. She left her story with me that afternoon, and I want to share her words with you.

My parents live in a small town on the South Dakota border about two hundred miles from where I live. They used to be farmers, and until fairly recently they lived in their own home. My mother is now ninety-two, and she suffers from dementia. My father is ninety. His mind is still sharp, but he has major physical limitations. He fell a couple of years ago and severely injured himself. He can't walk, he's incontinent, and he has very little energy. When it became difficult to find help to come to their home and to get them the nursing and personal services they needed, my four siblings and I thought it would be best for our parents to move into a nursing home. I found a good facility in the area where they've always lived. That's where they are now. I drive two hundred miles every weekend to visit them.

I guess you'd call me the primary caregiver. How did that happen, when I have four brothers and a sister? Two of my siblings say they are too busy with their jobs and families to make the time; the other two have told me that it's just too hard for them to deal with the situation emotionally or to travel to the care facility on a regular schedule. My sisters do visit, but not as regularly as I do. I guess the dynamics of every family are different. I've always felt close to my parents, and caregiving seemed the right thing for me to do. I just fell into the whole caregiving thing. It's now become a part of my lifestyle.

I began to go see my mother and father every weekend

before they went to live in the nursing home. I could see how valuable my efforts were to them. I would drive up on the weekend after work and stay with them until Sunday night. I'd do the cleaning and the shopping and whatever was necessary to take care of them. I worked on making their house more wheelchair accessible. I installed a shower, had a deck built, and tried to keep them comfortable in their home for as long as possible. Now I supervise their care in the nursing home, handle their financial matters, and care for their house. They no longer live in it, but I bring my mother out to stay in their home every weekend. My dad is in a wheelchair and needs a van to transport him. The local service isn't always available, but when it is, he comes out to the house too. He seems so tired; I think he's just shutting down. He's outlived his friends and everyone in his family. I know my mother is a real worry to him.

My mother loves flowers and was a dedicated gardener, so being at home gives her pleasure. It's my responsibility to keep up the garden so she'll have flowers to pick. Because she has a fear of falling, we plant the flowers in pots on the deck, so she can enjoy them without going down the hill. She likes to do things in the kitchen, like wash the dishes after I've been cooking. These are things she can't do in the nursing home, but they are familiar tasks she's been doing all her life. Even though she's senile, she can still do these kinds of things. My mother doesn't eat because she's hungry; she eats for social reasons. So I take her to a restaurant or to my aunt's house, or we use her favorite dishes and cups and set the table and linens to make a social environment at home. I feel these are important things to do for her.

My mother's moods are difficult. She has her ups and downs, and she's impatient about many things and demanding at times.

I keep learning how to handle it; things are constantly changing, of course. I'm pretty familiar with her behavior, though, and when she can't find the words I can pretty much tell what she's trying to communicate. I've come to understand that certain things are disturbing to people who are losing their ability to communicate. For example, sometimes three people will come into my parents' room in the nursing home—one handing her medication, one combing her hair, and another cleaning the room. It's just too much for her, and she gets very agitated. Mother doesn't hear well, but even if she hears, she can't always make sense of what everyone is saying. That's when she's uncooperative, and you've lost her for a while. She knows that I'm one of her children, but she doesn't know exactly who I am, and she's beginning to confuse generations.

My coming every weekend is a help to my father too. Although it's too hard for him to come with us to the house every weekend, it's a relief for him to know I'll be here to take care of my mother. And then, too, he knows the bills will be paid, the property will be taken care of, and nothing will be neglected. I've driven through snowstorms, heavy rain, and all kinds of weather to get there. I've never let them down.

I know that the schedule I've taken on to care for my parents could put a terrible stress on most marriages. But my husband and I have become closer, and we have come to understand each another better. My husband has been extremely supportive. I think he really admires what I'm doing. Sometime he comes with me, but it isn't always convenient for him. We joke that having a few days apart is good for our relationship.

There's great joy for me in bringing some happiness to my folks and to the other older people at the nursing home. I've struck up relationships with some of the other residents. We've become friends, and sometimes I even take one or two of them on an outing. I don't think the administration at the nursing home particularly likes it when I take people other than my mom out to lunch. I'm sure I'm breaking some rules. But you know what? I'm glad I have the courage to break some rules to make one day better for people who might live the rest of their lives in the nursing home. To give them some pleasure, to make them smile, to hear them laugh is so rewarding. I joke with one old farmer and always blame him for the weather. I bring in tractor books for a few of the older men who were farmers all their lives. It's really easy to make these older people glow! This isn't just about my giving my time and effort to others. I really get a lot of satisfaction and pleasure back.

Once I was talking with an elderly woman about birds or something, and pretty soon another lady came over and joined the conversation. Nearby was another woman just sitting in her wheelchair, totally motionless, stiff and unresponsive. As the three of us talked, I noticed this woman's wheelchair backing up, and before I knew it she was sitting in our circle listening to the conversation. I'm finding that this happens a lot. The people in this nursing home need that social connection, and when we all get to talking, they won't let me go!

I'd consider moving into my parents' house and living there except for my job. I work for a publisher and book distributor, and I love my work. I love books, and my mother also cares a lot about books. It's the one thing she remembers. When I tell her on Sunday night that I'm leaving so I can go to my office on Monday morning, she says, "Oh, what do you do? You work with books? Oh, how nice, that's nice work. You are so lucky to be with books." She worked in the local library for years, and she was an avid reader. Those things she remembers.

I've learned a lot about giving care, and I've also learned something about myself. A few days with my parents, and I'm ready to get back to my own life until the next weekend. I can do caregiving well, and I really enjoy it, but I need to take care of myself. Becoming a successful caregiver is a process of understanding your limitations.

Caregiving is probably the most rewarding thing I've ever done and also the most difficult. I know my mother probably doesn't remember the details of my visits, but I have the warm and wonderful experience of seeing her light up for that one minute when I arrive on the weekends. I think the smiles and laughs we share keep her healthier. Sometimes she responds to me in such a way that you'd never know she was senile. I'll say to her, "You know, you're my best mom," and she'll reply, "That's because I'm your only mom!" She smiles every time we have that exchange. It's the best feeling for me. It makes my day.

Long-distance caregiving has become a common phenomenon of our time. Grown children often move away from where their parents live because they go to college, accept a job offer, marry, or explore other options that can't be matched where their parents reside. Depending on a specific situation, some middle-aged and younger children are ready and willing to take on the challenge of a long-distance caregiving responsibility. Many years ago, when my childless aunt who lived alone after the death of her husband needed care, I accepted that responsibility from across the country. I jumped on an airplane every other weekend to go to my aunt's home to do what needed to be done and to meet with the persons hired to provide the practical everyday help. Each long-distance caregiver has his or her own individual story along with the stresses, compromises, and challenges that are part of accepting that role.

After her parents could no longer manage in their home, Ardith helped them move into a care residence not far from where they had always lived. Staff members tend to residents' practical and physical care. But often no one serves the interpersonal needs, tending to the casual, social interaction that people crave, no matter where they live.

I smiled when Ardith told me of taking others to lunch with her mom, including them in her conversations, and making time to talk with other residents at the nursing home. At the time of my interview with Ardith, the budget in many care establishments often didn't allow the facility to accommodate the social needs of residents whose relatives and longtime friends weren't living in the immediate area. I'm happy to say that many managers of facilities now recognize the importance of tending to the social needs of facility residents.

My conversation with Ardith brought up another important issue. Although Ardith was totally present during her weekend visit, she was eager and ready to get home to her husband and her job after the weekend. Both time with her husband and time for her work are important and satisfying parts of her life. Primary family caregivers often have to give up, modify, or temporarily put on hold things in their lives that are enjoyable in addition to jobs, children, and other commitments and obligations. However, whether work, classes, a hobby, or a regular exercise routine, such activities are important and need to remain part of a caregiver's life.

1. **I'm very aware that each long-distance caregiver's situation is different. There are no rules or formulas for this varied and challenging situation. Families do best when they discuss their situation together, when they make decisions on what each can do or is willing or able to contribute. I believe that caregiving needs require a family, large or small, to work out**

agreeable details and accept what specific responsibilities they can and are willing to accept.

2. What experiences have you had visiting a retirement residence where people are sitting around, not talking to one another, seeming isolated and noncommunicative? What have those times been like for you? How have you handled those situations? What changes might improve such situations?

3. Have you, or anyone you know, taken on a long-distance caregiver responsibility? How have decisions been made with your family or families you've worked with or counseled? How have the immediate families of the long-distance caregiver dealt with whatever responsibilities they've agreed to handle? How has family stress been resolved? What other reactions or consequences to the long distance caregiving situation have you had?

4. As there is no one right solution in a long-distance relationship for either the caregiver or the one in care, how might you suggest a family adjust to such a situation?

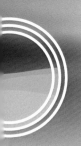

JULIAN

THERE'S NO PREDICTING

THE RECORDED MESSAGE ON MY ANSWERING MACHINE WAS from Julian. Although eighty-four years old, Julian still worked full time coaching, consulting, advising, and problem solving. "I'm not an authority on their specific business," he had once explained to me, "but I can help those I advise see how best to solve their problems. I deal with both little companies and big ones."

When we finally spoke, I quickly found out that his work wasn't the reason he had called. Julian had heard that I was seeking to talk with people who had been family caregivers and was eager to share his personal story. Julian invited me to look through hundreds of photographs he had taken of his wife, Thelma, over the seven-year period he cared for her. "As a tribute to her, I hope to mount a showing soon in cooperation with our local Alzheimer's group," he told me. "I think it's important for people to see how I loved and valued her even as the disease drained her energy, shrunk her stature, and changed who she was."

My experience as a caregiver started before I was even aware of it. Little changes had been taking place in Thelma's behavior for quite a while, but I didn't connect them with dementia at the time. She had macular degeneration, and we both were preoccupied with the changes in her eyesight. I guess I thought some of her behavior changes were because of these new limitations in her vision.

She had a habit of playing the piano every afternoon. Then, one day, she just couldn't do it. I thought it was because she was having trouble seeing the sheet music, so I made copies that were very large. They measured eighteen by twenty-four inches. She said she could see it fine but that her hands didn't know what to do anymore. I didn't realize that it was an early stage of deterioration in Thelma's thinking processes.

Once, we went to the supermarket where we'd shopped for more than thirty years. I left Thelma in the produce department while I went to pick up some other things on our list. When I came back I couldn't find her. I eventually spotted her wandering around, lost and agitated. I wanted to believe the cause was diminished eyesight, not mental deterioration, but eventually I took her to get some help. One doctor who was good in his diagnosis but extremely poor in his sensitivity sat us both down and blurted out, "Your wife has Alzheimer's."

Over the next few months Thelma's condition changed rapidly. She became depressed and more agitated. She paced around the house, and one day she bolted out and ran down the street. After that incident, I knew it was time to get some help with her care. There's a wonderful agency here in our town that focuses on the family member who is doing the caregiving. They sent someone over to help me understand how to manage the changing situation in our household, how to modify my work schedule so I could keep seeing a few clients, and, most important, how to take care of myself. I engaged helpers to come in from nine in the morning until six in the evening. I handled the nighttime alone for a while, but it was too difficult for me. That's when I had another person come in from seven in the evening to six in the morning.

My married son helped me organize the running of our household. That freed me up to spend more time with Thelma. Although the Thelma who I used to know wasn't fully there anymore, I wanted her to feel as much like herself as possible. We always dressed her in pretty clothes. I would spend time at the beach with her, because Thelma loved being near the ocean. My son and I would transfer her to her wheelchair and take her up into the hills too. She loved the outdoors.

I'd start every day helping the paid caregiver dress and bathe Thelma, and I'd be with her at breakfast and during the morning until she needed a nap. I was able to keep working almost every day until late in the afternoon. I needed the outside stimulation; it helped me keep balanced. When I came home, Thelma and I would have a little party. We'd sit in the living room and have ice cream and cake. It became our ritual.

Another thing that Thelma and I did together was share a story hour. I had a conversation with a caring and understanding librarian, and she suggested I read to Thelma from books written for ten- to twelve-year-old girls. Some people say that people with Alzheimer's can't focus on a story of any length, but I'm convinced they're wrong. One day when I was reading to Thelma, she was comfortable and relaxed, and I guess I must have been relaxed too. I don't remember falling asleep, but I do remember waking up and hearing Thelma say, "And then what happened?" She was still connected to the story.

The Alzheimer's group in town offered a two-day workshop for caregivers. During those two days, there was a session on learning the language of emotions. The leader of the group asked me to think of a time when I was sitting with Thelma. "Tell me what Thelma was saying to you." I told her that just yesterday we had sat together for quite a while, but Thelma didn't communicate anything, because she can use only a word or two, and those words usually don't have anything to do with what is going on right then. The leader asked, "Why don't you describe the expression that was on Thelma's face?" I was able to do that in some detail. Then she asked me to recall what was going on with her hands and feet, and to describe the look in Thelma's eyes and the expressions on her brow, prompting me, "What do you think Thelma was communicating?" I replied, "I guess she was telling me that she was feeling anxious, tense, and uncomfortable." I recalled that I kept asking her, "What do you want, Thelma? More ice cream? A pillow? A blanket? Are you cold? Are you too warm?" She gave no answer except more agitated movements of her hands and feet and a rather pained look in her eyes. Then the leader said, "So what if it happens again, how might you handle it differently?" I was silent for a long while. Then I got it. "Oh, I know. I'd just give her a hug."

Now, that's a long story about a simple thing. But for a man who is very logical, rational, and linear in the way he thinks, that was a profound learning experience. From that time on, although I didn't become highly skilled in emotional communication, I began to understand what was going on with Thelma's feelings. I also knew that whatever was going on inside her, she basically needed to feel safe, secure, and loved.

As things changed for Thelma, my life changed too. I realized that I was going through a learning process and that Thelma's illness was changing everything in my life. I remember that at one time, when things got difficult, I considered moving Thelma to a care facility and went to look at several. I decided I just couldn't separate from her. I was struggling with the decision, and a friend said to me, "Do you understand what this conflict you're having is all about? You want to have her with you no matter what. Thelma is the heart of your life." And he was right. I needed her as much as she needed me. That remark gave me a new understanding of our situation and was a great comfort.

People would tell me all the time how I was such a loving and caring companion, yet it was all very natural to me. Thelma would have done the same thing for me if our situations had been reversed. You know, I really got a lot back from what I gave. It may sound strange, but as I was losing Thelma, I began to understand love in a different way. We so often say the word *love*. We say it so easily without always knowing the feeling of love. Even as Thelma was growing more distant, I was feeling more deeply what love is. There was a mutual delight in our being together, a spiritual connection, a new feeling of love that I was just beginning to understand. In the midst of all I was losing, I began to know love in a way I had never experienced.

I understand and empathize with Julian's story about not recognizing Thelma's early symptoms of forgetting and confusion as the beginning of a more serious and progressive deterioration. It's something he didn't want to see or accept. Only when Thelma left the house unexpectedly and forgot where she was, even in familiar places, did Julian accept the sad reality as a sign of a problem. It's extremely difficult to adjust to such things in someone we love and share our life with. We instinctively resist recognizing symptoms that can mean huge changes and adjustments ahead in our lives.

Caring for a loved one with Alzheimer's disease or other progressive memory changes or confusion can require continual adjustments for both the family caregiver and others who visit. There's no predicting what might happen as each day passes. I've been present when others were also visiting a person with memory loss. I agree with the wisdom that Julian arrived at when Thelma was attempting to communicate. Offering a hug, an embrace, a kiss on the forehead, or just holding a hand says, "I'm here with you and for you."

1. Has anyone in your family or in your care as a professional been diagnosed with Alzheimer's disease or experienced other forgetting and confusion requiring care? How have members of the immediate family accepted the diagnosis? What help and support have others offered in these difficult situations?

2. Based on personal conversations, with groups of caregivers or with others who have now taken on such responsibilities, what do you think are the primary issues caregivers face when dealing with various stages of memory loss? From whom have they received advice and support?

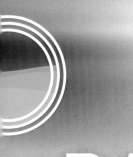

BARB

KEEPING CONNECTED

"YOUR NEW BOOK IS ABOUT FAMILY CAREGIVERS?" MY FRIEND Barb inquired. "Come on over, and we'll talk about that. I have a story to tell you. Caregiving is something we teach seriously and practice actively in my family."

When I arrived at Barb's house, she was sitting by the fireplace in her living room, composing a new melody on her guitar and singing words I hadn't heard before. "This is a new poem, one I've just written. I'll set it to music and sing it for you when it's finished. I can recite the poem for you today," she said.

Barb is a singer, songwriter, music educator, and performer. I've heard her share her music for both children and adults. Barb specializes in events that mark life passages: memorial services, funerals, bar mitzvahs, birth ceremonies. In describing her career Barb said, "As a musician I see myself as part of events that bring families and communities together. As a teacher, an educator, and artist, I try to capture personal memories and special feelings." Now it was my turn to collect personal memories and special feelings about caregiving experiences in her family.

My aunt Carol died two months ago at the age of eighty-eight. She'd been in a nursing home for almost ten years, diagnosed with Alzheimer's. I was there the day she died. She was agitated. I sat with her, held her hand, talked to her, and sang.

We take care of each other in our family. It's just how we function. For a long time, my mother took care of everyone in the family who was ill. She was always there for others. When my mother died three years ago, I felt I should take over for her as the primary caregiver. I knew that if she were still alive, she'd be doing this for others in the family. I felt it was my responsibility to take over.

I sort of drifted into being the contact for Aunt Carol's care in the Alzheimer's unit she was living in. I went to her care conferences at the nursing home and kept in touch with her dietician, physical therapist, and others responsible for her care. Aunt Carol's husband, my uncle Bert, helped for a while. Then he became rather frail and needed help from the family too. Six of us cousins in the younger generation formed a web of support around both Aunt Carol and Uncle Bert. My brother took charge of the main care for Uncle Bert—his bills and some personal care.

I recall how hard it was for Uncle Bert to put Aunt Carol in the nursing home. He wanted to be there with her all the time. They had been married for more than sixty years, and their relationship was one of deep and abiding love.

When Uncle Bert's health started to fail, he moved into an assisted living facility. I would pick him up and take him to see Aunt Carol as often as I could. I sensed the deep connection between them, and I wanted to honor that. Spending time with Aunt Carol and Uncle Bert gave me the time and opportunity to observe a love story. When I brought Uncle Bert to visit Aunt Carol, I'd walk away for a while so they could have their own time and space together. Although they were sitting together in wheelchairs in a room full of other people, I wanted them to have a feeling of privacy.

One day when I brought Uncle Bert to visit Aunt Carol, she was in a grumpy, distant mood. Yet, after a short time I saw her reach out, touch his hand, and gently start stroking his arm. I watched as a soft, loving look came over her face. It brought tears to my eyes to watch them. It was incredibly beautiful for me to see that even if she might not have recognized him at first, she knew him by touch. They were truly connected. Observing this taught me a lot about love and about family relationships and how deep that goes.

My way of expressing my thoughts and feelings is to put them on paper as poetry and then compose music for their presentation to others. My personal stories and experiences have become part of my performance repertoire. Inspired by Aunt Carol and Uncle Bert's lifelong relationship, I've just written a poem that I call "Where Love Resides." Even when you read the words without music, I think it speaks to the heart. I love to tell their story and share it with others.

Barb asked me, "Can I share it with you now?" "Yes, of course," I replied. "I want to know more about how, in spite of dementia, aging, and loss, love survives."

Where Love Resides

One single tear spills down my cheek
I am struck
Thinking how tragic, how sad
That after a lifetime of loving each other
It comes down to this
Sitting together,
Side by side
Wheelchair to wheelchair
Holding hands
That's all there is, nothing more
I've brought him to see her again
To the Oasis unit
Locked ward of the nursing home
For those on the steady downward slope
Of Alzheimer's decline
You can't get out the door unless you know the code
Can't get out of this disease at all
No one knows that code
We sit with sunlight streaming in the windows
This big room is peaceful and calm today
Other times, residents have wandered by
Shouting or swearing
"Take me home! Bring me back!"
"Where's my furniture? Where's my kitchen?"
"I want my mother."
But today is different
This lounge is quiet, tranquil
No one crying out, no moaning
No loud voices talking to thin air,
To a long-gone lover or friend, daughter or son
A forgotten argument in some long-ago time
No one moving in that slow solo dance

Within fragments of old memories
We sit, with me on his left
He is in the middle, she is on his right
I am drifting in memories myself
Of childhood gatherings, laughter, and loving faces
My grandma and my grandpa
My mom and my dad
Who've all passed on now
Sweet memories alive, but only in my heart
I think about this aunt and this uncle I sit with today
Both in their eighties, married almost sixty years
She seems oblivious, very much inside herself
Barely smiles when we first sit down
Staring ahead with a kind of sour look on her face
Doesn't recognize me as her niece, or him as her husband
Those days seem past
Since she could look at him and call him by his name
Long time since we've been able to sit
And talk about the same thing, or anything
Even have a conversation grounded
In the same perceived present reality
Sometimes she'll talk in half-formed sentences
Words strung together in ways
I can barely follow or understand
Fleeting memories bobbing in and out of a crazy quilt of time.
Another silent tear rolls down my cheek as I muse in the sunlight
Bittersweet—a lifetime of loving condensed
Into a passing moment together
He reaches out and takes her hand as he often does when we visit
Sometimes she quietly holds his hand, too
But today is different
This day, as he holds her hand
She slowly starts to squeeze his back
Then she strokes it, and her face changes

Smiling, she says, "Oh, oh, oh"
She touches his fingers, his thumb, and the back of his hand
She says, "This is nice,"
As though her skin recognizes his
Her mind can't say his name, but her body knows him
Memory and love living bone deep
She touches his hand, his arm
His shirt sleeve, and says again,
"This is nice!"
He says, "Oh yes, I like this shirt, it's a good shirt"
She sits back, her hand holding his
Her whole face transformed
With a gentle, sweet, contented smile
It is amazing to be together in this rare moment
Sharing the same intersection of time and space
One single tear spills down my cheek
I am struck
Thinking how incredible, how profoundly beautiful
That, after a lifetime of loving each other
It all comes down to this
Sitting together
Side by side
Wheelchair to wheelchair
In their holding hands
The heart bridges the gap
The mind alone cannot leap
Where touch knows touch
Skin knows skin
And love resides cell-deep
Weaving memory and connection

© Barb Tilsen. Used with permission.

My caregiving experience with Aunt Carol has profoundly affected my sense of parenting and the importance of family connection. I brought my children to visit Aunt Carol and Uncle Bert. I wanted them to see that we take care of each other and that the generations of family are connected in this way. Caring for Aunt Carol and Uncle Bert has taught us what it really means to be a family. Uncle Bert tells other people, "No one has great nieces and nephews like I have." I tell him, "Uncle Bert, in letting us care for you and Aunt Carol, you taught us that." My grandparents, my parents—they all did it for each other, so it only feels natural that we should be doing this too. Being a caregiver has deepened the ways I think about love, family, and commitment. It hasn't been a burden for me. It's been a deep, personal journey—a very special experience.

Barb describes caring connections with extended family members that don't widely exist these days. We rarely hear of family members still living close enough to physically connect easily. Because Barb and her aunt and uncle live in the same city, taking her uncle to visit his wife in a nursing home presents no problem. How rare this is in many family situations these days. We so often hear of close relatives taking airplanes or trains to accomplish such visits and sustain connections. The needs exist, but the solution isn't always simple.

I hope families will recognize family members' needs and, no matter how far away they live, make arrangements to visit and keep connected with their loved ones living in senior residences, receiving medical care, or adjusting to new environments.

Some responsibilities of family caregiving include providing transportation to regularly visit a loved one; to maintain connections with close, perhaps sick or disabled, friends and others; to go to medical appointments; and even to go shopping. Some people won't ask for help. It's wise for someone in the family to stay aware of the changes and needs of the elders and, as appropriate, to step in and address their personal situations.

1. Are you aware of a family member or someone you know through work connections who needs transportation for medical appointments, visits to friends, grocery shopping, or other needs?

2. You might be aware of people who need help but are reluctant to ask. How can someone in the family or circle of acquaintances keep track of the events and connection in that person's life and offer transportation or other help as needs become evident?

3. When has offering transportation to someone who no longer drives made possible an important visit or an event? Share that story and what you've learned from that experience.

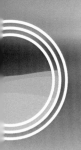

CAROL

A GIFT IN DISGUISE

DIVORCED, WITH TWO GROWN CHILDREN, CAROL WAS LIVING alone and building an interesting and rewarding consulting career while enjoying an active social life. Like many children of aging parents, Carol lived almost three thousand miles from her eighty-year-old mother, who lived alone and refused to move from her very old, two-story house that was in need of repair. For as long as Carol could remember, her mother, who had been widowed for more than fifty years, had been an incredibly strong, independent woman, but Carol was aware that that her mom's strength and health were slowly deteriorating.

Carol monitored her mother's health and daily activity as diligently as the distance and commitments to her job and personal life allowed. She called her mom on the phone five or six times a day. She flew from California to New Jersey six or seven times a year, bought two months worth of groceries at a time, cooked individual meals, and filled the freezer. She also cleaned the house and organized her mother's affairs as best she could. Then she'd fly home and again phone her mom numerous times a day to be sure she was okay. This pattern continued for a number of years.

Carol was fifty-two when I had a conversation with her. A year had passed since the death of her mother. Carol and I sat together drinking tea and reflecting on her caregiving experience. She talked about how she had decided to handle all her mother's needs and what she had learned from her experience. Carol began telling her story before I even asked a question.

It was stressful, I'll tell you. One summer I went back to New Jersey with a plan to spend the summer with Mother. I thought I'd certainly be coming back to California in the fall, but I had to face the reality that she was getting weaker and weaker. I came to the conclusion that it was better for me to put my life in California on hold and go stay with her. I knew I could no longer deal with the stress and frustration of being a long-distance caregiver. I finished up my consulting contracts, gave notice on the house I was renting, put virtually everything I owned in storage, packed up what I needed, and moved across the country and settled down in her house.

At first I felt alone and missed the life I had left behind. But gradually I began to take hold of my new situation. I found the neighbors to be some of the dearest, sweetest, finest people I'd ever met, the salt of the earth. They were incredibly supportive of me during the last eighteen months of my mother's life.

I reconnected with cousins, my last remaining uncle, and other members of my family. That was a bonus I hadn't counted on. I felt love and support from each neighbor, relative, and old friend. It was truly a beautiful and unexpected experience.

I realized that I couldn't cure Mother, but I could work on healing myself. There I was sleeping in the bed I had slept in when I was eight years old, preparing meals on the stove I had learned to cook on when I was ten. I spent time walking the streets of the town I had grown up in, past the homes where relatives and friends once lived, past the church I had been married in and the school I had attended from kindergarten through the tenth grade. It became a time of healing a lot of the issues related to the death of my father when I was very young. I was dealing with feelings of sadness and grief that I never imagined I would revisit, much less resolve and heal.

My relationship with my mother had always been good. But now we became deeply, deeply close. Over those eighteen months of caregiving, I learned so much about death and dying. It was a powerful, intense, in-the-trenches education in caregiving. I was experiencing the psychological side of it, the spiritual side of it, and the physical side of it. I took on bathing her, cleaning her, looking for miracles, putting everything I had into trying to keep her alive.

Now I hardly remember the hard parts. It might sound strange, but I only remember the good stuff. I remember how wonderful it was to slow down and just sit on her old couch on snowy afternoons and listen to her. I remember going out to dinner with friends and coming home at midnight and finding her sitting on the sofa at eighty-nine just the way she did when I was nineteen years old, saying to me, "I was so worried about you. How can you do this to me? How can you make me worry about you?" It was really adorable to have my mom still care that much. Other people might freak out and say, "Mom, I'm over fifty years old!" But I was deeply touched, because I knew that soon she wouldn't be sitting on that sofa anymore. Those final years when people are slipping away from us can be so precious.

My mother was fading, but at least I didn't have the stress of dealing with someone who is dying of cancer or in constant pain. When she experienced her last bout of congestive heart failure, I took her to the hospital and she slipped into a coma. I said to the doctor, "What's happening here?" The doctor said, "She'll linger like this for five or six days. There's nothing more we can do." And I said, "I want to take her home to die where she'd want to be."

I quickly realized that I couldn't do it alone. A caregiver has to have a helpmate in this process. Everyone needs some respite in these situations. I was blessed to have a wonderful companion caregiver who had helped me care for Mother the previous few months. The two of us brought her home and put her in her bed of sixty-seven years and brushed her hair and put on the prettiest nightgown we could find. Then we sat with her for three days and held her hand. And one night she just stopped breathing.

So, it had been eighteen months of caregiving, laughing, crying, hugging, sharing, going over photographs, and celebrating holidays. Yes, sometimes we argued and were impatient with each other. I was terrified as she declined physically, but somehow I found the strength and the courage to let her go.

Looking back on those months, I feel it's important to tell you what I learned. Caring for my mother helped me face something I had managed to avoid before: thinking about death, about mortality, and about how fragile we humans are. We're here for only a little while. We need to let those around us know that we love them and care about them, that they matter to us. I pay attention to this now. I let my family and friends know they are important in my life. When I think about those conversations with my mother I know they were gifts I never would have experienced from afar. Through taking care of my dying mother, I learned not only about facing death and dying but also about the value of each day of living.

In spite of the sadness with the death of her mother and the move across country that demanded a total change in her personal and work life, Carol found the rewards were unexpected and deeply satisfying. Living independently and being divorced, with her children grown and on their own, she was able to make that decision. Some family members make plane trips two or three times a month to supervise the care of a loved one, because they aren't able to move. Some are often obliged to leave behind husbands and children and get temporary leave from work to care for a loved one. We make whatever compromises are possible or necessary and modify them as situations change. However, the personal growth and deep satisfaction growing out of Carol's decision to become an on-location caregiver offered unexpected intimacy for both her mother and her—a gift in disguise.

There are no right or wrong ways to assume a commitment to family caregiving. Carol's decision proved to be rewarding and satisfying for her and her mother. It was obviously the right decision for Carol. I've kept in touch with her, and she has told me of many helpful and thoughtful conversations she's had since her mother's death with others facing long-distance family care challenges.

1. Have you or others you know been responsible for the care of someone in a long-distance situation? How can support

be offered to someone who can't move? How can you offer support to a long-distance caregiver for whatever decisions he or she makes?

2. What stories are you aware of about neighbors and friends who supported a caregiver? Have you ever been in such circumstances? What might an active and involved neighbor or friend learn from the experience?

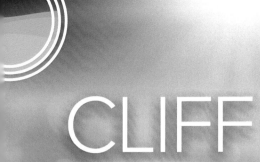

CLIFF

THE VALUE OF EACH MOMENT

THEIR YEARS OF BUILDING CAREERS WERE OVER. IT WAS TIME TO travel, explore new interests and hobbies, and enjoy life. Cliff was a therapist who saw clients in his office adjacent to their spacious suburban home. Cathy was active, friendly, and well liked. We had become friends, and I looked forward to our times together. Her conversation was informed, thoughtful, bright, and witty. Being with her was fun.

One day Cathy discovered a small lump in her breast. She went to the doctor immediately; although he was reassuring, the doctor suggested it might be wise to have a biopsy. This story is not about recovery from cancer but about a beautiful relationship that grew deeper as Cathy's illness progressed. Cliff talked with me about the woman he loved and lost. He was silent, looking out of a nearby window as I waited until he began telling his story.

I remember very clearly the day Cathy told me the results of the biopsy. She had breast cancer. Everything followed soon—surgery, decisions about chemotherapy, a follow-up that revealed another lump, more surgery, and more chemotherapy. It seemed endless.

Through it all, I came to understand at a profound level that it was vital to find ways to deal with such things. I developed a new understanding for ways of coping that are often described as denial. You need to develop an open and accepting frame of mind of the real situation in order to deal with serious illness. You must find ways of surviving and of holding yourself together, dealing with what comes next, taking care of yourself, and supporting the person you're caring for. That requires not just what people blithely refer to as building up defenses. Each person figures out how to handle his or her situation.

I think we were realistic about the severity of Cathy's illness, but we also knew we had to have hope. The one thing that was hopeful for me was uncertainty. All through my wife's illness, even when her cancer reoccurred after a period of remission, I still clung to the hope that perhaps, statistically, she would be in the most fortunate category. I guess what happens is that gradually the circle of hope narrows and narrows. For us, it was during the summer of the year she would die that we both really knew there weren't many options left.

It was the end of the summer, and we were closing up our vacation home. Usually when we locked it up, we anticipated returning the following spring. But this time we both knew that was not going to happen. I remember the last day we walked on the beach together. We were aware that this was the last time we'd take this walk together. It was a terribly sad day and the first of many experiences through this whole process that we knew we would never again share.

We were about to leave the beach, and both Cathy and I were on the edge of weeping when we bumped into some neighbors who were chattering away. It was like a scene out of a movie, those people talking and talking at a moment that was for us so poignant and painful. Paradoxically, it somehow helped us. I didn't know how we were going to leave the beach that day, a place of so many memories, so many summers together, so many times walking together, picking up seashells, playing with our children, and sharing our lives. It was terribly painful, yet we had to face it, and we didn't quite know how. Somehow this chattering couple enabled us to get through it. I saw it as a blessing. I think we would have just collapsed otherwise.

That fall we knew Cathy was approaching the end. The oncologist told us about another new drug they were testing and suggested we consider more chemotherapy. It was then that, together, we consciously chose a different path. We had gone through enough. The treatment had become the illness; it had become worse than the disease. We decided that Cathy would not have any further treatments, and that had a very positive effect. It was sad, but we felt somehow that we were in control and her illness was no longer managing us. We knew now that whatever time was left, we would have it together.

We became as close as two human beings could possibly become. When I look back, it is a time I really cherish. I'm so grateful we had that together. We spent a lot of time reviewing our lives together—the good things, the joys, and the fullness of it all. We talked about everything. Cathy and I had a very good marriage, a wonderful marriage, but like all marriages it also had some rough spots. We had done or said some mean, thoughtless things to each other in the past, as couples often do. Now we had an opportunity to come to some peace about those things. We forgave each other for the rough times we had given one another. It was very important that we had the time and the wisdom to do this.

Cathy also told me she wanted me to marry again. Part of me felt guilty about even thinking of remarrying. It seemed like a betrayal. But I knew she was being honest. Cathy didn't want my loneliness and suffering to be her legacy. I sincerely believe she wanted me to remarry. I felt I had her blessing. It was to honor her spirit that I did go on with my life and eventually marry again.

Of course, a large part of me wishes Cathy were still here in my life. Her death was an enormous blow to me. I was really wiped out for quite a while. Some of my friends who had also lost a spouse told me that you never really get over it, and I've found that to be true. You never get over missing someone who was important to you, and that knowledge sits side by side with the new relationship.

I feel very blessed that I eventually met a woman who was able to understand and accept that. It actually was a number of years later that Judith came into my life. I don't feel that she and Cathy are in competition with each other. They each have their place in my life. I can miss Cathy, and I certainly do, and still enjoy being with the woman to whom I'm married now. She and I are able to talk about that. It's been important in our marriage. I don't know how I could have managed a new relationship otherwise.

The experience of Cathy's illness and death has made me better able to be with other people who are experiencing pain.

In my work as a therapist, I'm much more available now to people who are suffering or facing death. I know we can't always relieve pain and suffering, but we can be with other people, stay with them, be available to them, and not abandon them. I never realized how much I tended to withdraw from people in pain. We can't make some circumstances different, but we can stay with each other and support each other. I've learned to do this in a way that never would have been possible for me before. That's one way I've changed and grown from the experience of Cathy's death.

Another significant thing I've learned through all this is about time. Oh sure, I knew it intellectually, but now I know it in a fuller, more profound way. What I mean is I've come to understand that the most important thing we possess is time. I began learning that during Cathy's illness. We created more time for each other. I worked less, we spent more time alone together, we both learned to think about time in a different way, and I still do.

When you really know that your time will come to an end, when you're aware of death, I think you value time in a different way. It's the one thing you have control over, how you spend your time. This awareness has carried over into my life now. I continually ask myself, "Is this how I want to use the time that's left in my life?" I see clearly the areas of my life where I have control—and what things I can't control. I think of the phrase "living more fully," and that's what I do now. I learned from dealing with Cathy's illness and death how to live more consciously and with more awareness.

I've never before talked with someone who put as much of his or her work and independent life aside to spend time with a loved one whose life was ending. To talk about past misunderstandings, find a new depth of their love for each other, and to honestly discuss the survivor's remarrying was for each of them a deeply meaningful experience.

I've heard so many people express regret about not seeing someone before the person died to clear up old misunderstandings, to deepen their relationship, or about not making time to be together, knowing that soon it would not be possible. Cliff's story might speak to us all.

I was also struck by his observations about time, a precious commodity that in our fast-moving culture we risk not understanding. Some wonder, where did the time go? Didn't the summer go by much too fast? How can it possibly be her eightieth birthday? Because Cliff knew that Cathy's life was limited, he gained a new understanding of time and the value of each day that can remind us all of the real value of each moment.

1. A major focus on a diagnosis of a serious illness is treatment and cure and at least an attempt at prolonging life. Do you know of any situation where the ill person made the decision to give up treatment? How did the family respond? How did the ill person deal with the decision in the face of objections and suggestions?

2. Has an experience in your personal or work life brought you to a new and unexpected awareness of time? How has this concept filtered into your work or personal life? Have you brought the subject of time into a conversation, or might you consider doing that in the future? Why or why not?

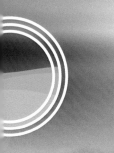

SHILA

SEEDS OF GROWTH

IF I HAD MET SHILA AND MORRIE FIVE YEARS EARLIER, I WOULD have thought that this attractive, smartly dressed couple had it all: a glamorous lifestyle, easy travel to exotic destinations, everything that money can offer. But material wealth is no guarantee against the ravages of illness, dementia, and loss. Shila and Morrie are both past midlife now. Morrie was diagnosed with Alzheimer's disease, and Shila has the responsibility of his care. When she shared her story with me, it was a powerful reminder that privilege doesn't protect one from pain. "I know I'm blessed with the ability to pay for around-the-clock care for my husband, yet I also know that money doesn't solve all the problems one is faced with when illness changes everything in your life." Through Morrie's illness Shila has found a wisdom that money just can't buy.

Morrie is my fourth husband. Finally I got it right! Before his illness, we traveled, enjoyed our life, and loved each other dearly. It was a life fully realized for me. He is, and always will be, the love of my life.

I really don't remember when the symptoms began. I guess it was about five and a half years ago. When I first consulted the doctors, they said, "No problem, just some little ministrokes. We can take care of that with medication, and he won't have any more." But no medication seemed to help, and the deterioration continued.

In August of that year, we went on what turned out to be our last vacation. We flew to Alaska to take a cruise for what we had hoped would be a wonderful two-week trip. But it didn't turn out that way. The whole time Morrie was confused, had trouble with understanding directions, and behaved unpredictably. I was so frightened that I couldn't let myself see what was happening. My denial was total. But when Morrie became unpredictably violent, there was no denying that something was terribly wrong.

He started having trouble with numbers, and that was extremely disturbing to him. Morrie has always been involved in high finance and big business. His life was crunching numbers. Suddenly it seemed all he would talk about was money. The reality is that we are very well off financially, and there was no basis for his concern. Maybe he was remembering that he was born to poor Greek immigrants. His father was a flower peddler who roasted nuts to supplement the family income. Morrie's dream was to have a fruit stand of his own. He got his fruit stand, and it was the beginning of what eventually became an empire.

Now that wealth supports his around-the-clock care. Of course, I'm aware that with the totally incapacitating illness my husband has, the money has been an enormous advantage. Financial security has assured paid professional caregiving that makes an enormous difference. I'm blessed that I don't have the stress and worries so many people do, but privilege doesn't take away the pain.

Morrie is severely demented now. We call it Alzheimer's, but that's one of a wide range of memory-related conditions. I've engaged warm, caring, competent people who take wonderful care of my husband. The violence that Morrie displayed at the onset isn't there anymore. The best medical advice we got was simply to stay out of verbal conflict with him, always to assure him he's right and that we'll do things his way. His short-term memory is so bad he doesn't remember what he said anyway. We keep him calm and happy, and, whatever is going on in his brain, he thinks he's in control and doesn't feel threatened. Morrie doesn't respond well to care from a man, so now the entire staff I employ is female. I think he sees a man as a challenge, and he puts up a fight. The nurses call him Papa Morrie, and they can get this big, strapping man to do whatever they ask. I call the staff his angels.

During the first two years of Morrie's decline I was physically ill, emotionally distraught, sleep deprived, hysterical, and on the edge of a nervous breakdown. For myself I tried medications, chiropractic, homeopathy, and acupuncture. All the things I tried at the physical level only gave me temporary relief. Psychotherapy and meditation were the two things that eventually enabled me to look for connections in the outside world that offered me comfort, peace of mind, and purpose.

That's when, through an acquaintance, I was introduced to the Science of Mind Church. It now has become my spiritual community. Although my cultural identification is with the Jewish religion, it was the friendship and support of the people at that church that helped me reach the acceptance of what is, rather than being stuck in what could have been. I've learned that what matters is not what life deals you, but what you do with the hand you've been dealt. I've received an abundance of loving guidance and new learning. I've turned my potential victimhood into what I've labeled "victorhood." I've come to understand that today is all we have and this moment is what we have now.

My church has given me a way to reach out and help many other people in need. I've found great comfort and satisfaction in giving money anonymously to help children and single mothers. I remember when I was raising two children alone, and many people did nice things for me without ever asking for anything in return. Now it's my turn to give. I give of myself and I give of my abundance. Thankfully, I've discovered that being able to give is the most selfish pleasure in the world.

I know that I've made a difference by helping others. I've found a way to consider Morrie's illness a gift, an opportunity to grow and expand, to genuinely share, and to help myself by helping others. Today my goals are to experience deeper spiritual growth and use my time and energy in outward service. I'm creating a rich and full life for myself. Certainly I have my sadness, but comfort comes from the quality of the life I'm leading and the people I've surrounded myself with. I feel a special energy from those around me. In spite of the tragedy of Morrie's illness, I truly believe my life is one of grace and blessing.

There have been many unexpected healings for me that have come out of Morrie's illness. At one time I resented that

Morrie's daughters didn't come to see him very often. I knew they felt mistrustful and frightened of me, and I of them. I had spent a lot of time being angry and resentful. That's all in the past. I've learned a lot about forgiveness. My negative feelings have been transformed into love and compassion. And that's the greatest gift I've gotten out of this sad situation.

One daughter who lives out of town comes to visit now at least once a month, sometimes more if her husband has business in town. The other one who lives here doesn't come that often. A few years ago I would have sat here with vitriol pouring out of me in resentment. Now I realize what a hard time she must have seeing her father like this, and I have to respect her decisions about what she feels she can handle. I've forgiven myself for making judgments, and that has allowed me to forgive her. Morrie's son who lives out of town has told me he just can't come very often. It's too hard for him to see his father this way. I respect and accept his decision too. He's been kind and supportive. So, I'm doing my best to get along in this world, and I believe they're doing the same. I'd say this change in my perspective is the most important gift I've had out of all this.

Morrie is seventeen years older than I am, so barring something unforeseen, he will probably die before me. It's interesting that I've already been through what I call the widow syndrome, where everybody comes around for a few weeks or months and then they disappear. I've already had the people fall away who weren't going to be with me for the long haul. If—I mean *when*—Morrie dies, I will grieve deeply. I know I'll be bereft for a time, but I won't have to ask myself, "What will I do with the rest of my life?" I'm living the rest of my life right now. Mostly I live in a state of gratitude for the ability to maintain him with every advantage. It's ironic, but as Morrie diminishes and his path becomes more and more limited, I'm expanding and growing my path.

My relationship with my husband is no longer anything like it was. I'm interchangeable with the nurses who take care of him. I haven't been able to lie down next to him for a long time. It's extremely painful for me. Only rarely do I cry now, but when I do, the tears pour out. But then it's over. Maybe it's sadness for what could have been or for who Morrie used to be, yet I know there's no benefit in pursuing that kind of thinking. Of course, it's distressing each time I see Morrie hit a new low, but I guess I've learned to adjust to those changes. The immediate feelings of fear and panic now pass quickly. I consciously choose not to look ahead and anticipate what will happen next.

Morrie and I are soul mates. I believe that, and I remember that although he isn't the person I used to know, my husband is still alive. I get to go in and kiss him, see that wonderful smile and the twinkle in his eye, and feel his warmth. I know that I'm truly, truly blessed.

When someone has the assurance of financial security or even abundance and is part of the financially privileged 1 percent, it's easy to think that person's challenges in dealing with a loved one's illness and decline are vastly different from the experience of those who are less fortunate. Shila viewed her own circumstance as a "gift" and welcomed the opportunity to grow and help herself by helping others.

Shila is not the first person I've heard talk about a relationship formed in later life that has brought a depth of love never before experienced. Yes, Shila was in her fourth marriage. For many, just that fact may overshadow what she has to say. However, I choose to believe that change and growth is possible for each of us and that Shila has used a sad situation to become a person she never knew before.

We all want to make a difference—to enrich and explore our personal lives and to make a contribution in our community, church or synagogue, or neighborhood. Unanticipated negative situations may also provide the seeds of growth and discovery that can offer new learning and understanding.

1. What other stories have you heard about a caregiver's growth, new insights, and positive changes in how the person is now living his or her life?

2. Shila reacted to her husband's dementia and erratic behavior by becoming physically ill, emotionally distraught, and sleep deprived, approaching a complete breakdown. How have others you know about or have witnessed found a path out of such self-destructive behaviors and feelings?

3. When have you experienced or witnessed resistance to and denial of a loved one's decline that eventually changed into a more realistic and accepting behavior?

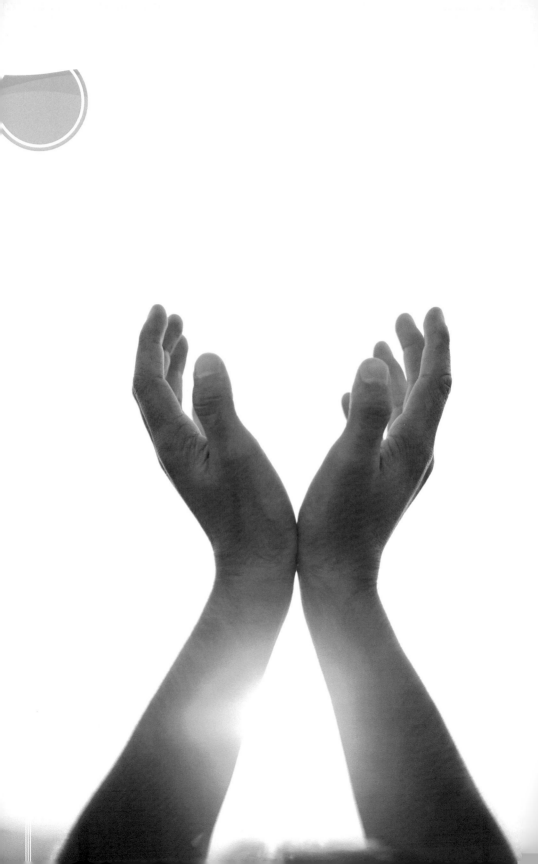

CYNTHIA

FEEDING MY SOUL

CYNTHIA GREW UP ON A FARM, THE ELDEST OF FIVE. SHE IS MAR-
ried, has two teenage children, and still lives on a farm. "I'm just
an ordinary person," she told me when we talked, but I found her
most extraordinary. She has worked as an interior designer, an
acting coach, and a professional model, but her passion is to help
and encourage others to be the best they can be in whatever
field of work or lifestyle they choose. Her self-described mission
is "to help you to recognize your individual gifts and tap into your
creative energies, so you can sparkle and soar in every area of
your life." Her inspiration to give this to others came from her dad.
She calls him her angel.

M y dad was my hero. He was incredibly caring; he
loved his wife and his children more than anything
in the world. We were all stars in his eyes. One day
my sister called me and said, "Cynthia, Daddy is dying." She
was hysterical. Dad had started throwing up blood; the doctor
suspected a rare form of cancer, leiomyosarcoma. My dad had
no symptoms except maybe heartburn. Because we're Italian

and we eat lots of spicy food, my father wasn't concerned about symptoms of indigestion. He had never been sick a day in his life. Now I was being told that the doctors had given him only three weeks to live.

I thought about all the times my dad had been there for me. I began calling every doctor I knew; I called around the country and found the most respected experts on this kind of cancer. I was absolutely shameless in asking for help. If the doctors were right and he only had a few weeks to live, I had to act fast. I kept hoping, even though I was told over and over again that a cancer that large could not be operated on and nothing could be done. Even if a cure wasn't possible, I thought maybe I could find a way to get some time. I guess I really believe miracles happen to those who also trust in them, people like me.

The first miracle was that I found a doctor who thought there was a chance with surgery. Then we received another miracle. The surgery gave my father a few more years of quality life. He went back to his ranch, planted a vineyard, installed an irrigation system, finished building a dam, and took a number of trips. Three years later the cancer came back with ferocity. At this point I realized we couldn't look toward a cure. The cancer had metastasized, and Daddy knew that he was dying. I told him I would be there with him until the very last breath. It was both the most difficult time and the most rewarding experience of my life.

My dad's last days truly were a gift. When he died, there were absolutely no regrets. Those three years that were supposed to be three weeks had given both him and me the time to realize the beauty of life. We experienced deeply how much we really loved each other, and we didn't hesitate to say it. I came to understand during that time that we only have this moment. I was able to say to my dad, "You are a gift and I love you. Thank you for all you've done. You've made a difference in my life, you've made a difference in the community, and you've made a difference in the world just by your being."

In the final weeks I stayed close to my dad and we talked a great deal. One day he smiled at me and said, "I'm dying a happy man. I married the woman I love and have shared forty-five years with her. I have five fabulous children, and I was blessed to be a farmer. It was my passion. I tilled the soil, and what I did fed people. I've lived my dream." What he said gave me a profound insight. This simple man, a salt-of-the-earth farmer, felt he had lived his destiny, his purpose, his dream. I thought, "Why are so many of us striving to be something we aren't in this world, struggling to fulfill someone else's idea of success, someone else's dream?" At that moment, my whole life changed. I realized that it was vital for each of us to truly be who we are, who we were born to be, to be the star we are—to find that light that shines within us and help that light shine brightly.

When my dad died, his last words to me were, "My end is your beginning." It was true. Since then I've created and hosted a television program called *Be the Star You Are*. It's about people who are doing what they love, not for the money, not for the glamour, but because they choose to do what feeds their soul. I really didn't know anything about producing a television show, so it's nothing short of a miracle that I was able to find people who supported my efforts and helped me broadcast twenty-eight episodes. For the most part, all the people I interviewed on the program were ordinary people who had followed their passion and fulfilled their dream. I had very little money to do the show, but somehow I found volunteers to donate their time and energy. I actually paid my camera crew with vegetables from my garden and fresh chicken eggs! I didn't do this program for money; it was my gift to others. I dedicated the series to my dad, who had been my inspiration. I've recently written a book called *Be the Star You Are! 99 Gifts for Living, Loving, Laughing, and Learning to Make a Difference.* I wrote it with love. I want to inspire others, and I know now that I can do that.

I treasure those years of my dad's illness even as I remember how difficult they were. Being able to care for him and to help was such a joy, because it was in that time that I learned the meaning of life. I learned that it doesn't matter how many awards you win, how many trophies you have, how much money you've made. There's only one thing at the end of the day and at the end of our lives that matters, and that is love— loving and respecting yourself and showing others that you care about them. Loving is how we really make a difference. My dad taught me that. He was my teacher, my angel, and my hero.

I suspect that too often we pay attention primarily to the inconveniences emerging from a situation. For many people a caregiving job is to be done "because my family needs my help, and then I'll go back to my life as it was." But taking on a family caregiving role may inspire new thinking about our choices for the future. Cynthia's caregiving experience with her father, that unanticipated relationship, led her to embrace a new direction. It was the seed of a career of service that she never planned or expected.

I've come to believe that unexpected events that first appear threatening or negative can, with a different point of view, become the seeds of growth. Cynthia's story may offer us another way to understand and act on what many people would see as a negative event. Of course, the death of Cynthia's beloved father was an experience of loss and sadness, but growth can come at unexpected times.

1. In your family, or with any of your clients, have you followed up with the caregiver survivor to ask about the person's learning, growth, or changes in his or her life arising from the caregiving experience? In reflection, what does the caregiver say he or she has learned or in what ways may it have changed the person's life?

2. Have you had a personal caregiver experience that has resulted in new learning and important changes in your life? What can you share that will open discussions with others about such unexpected growth?

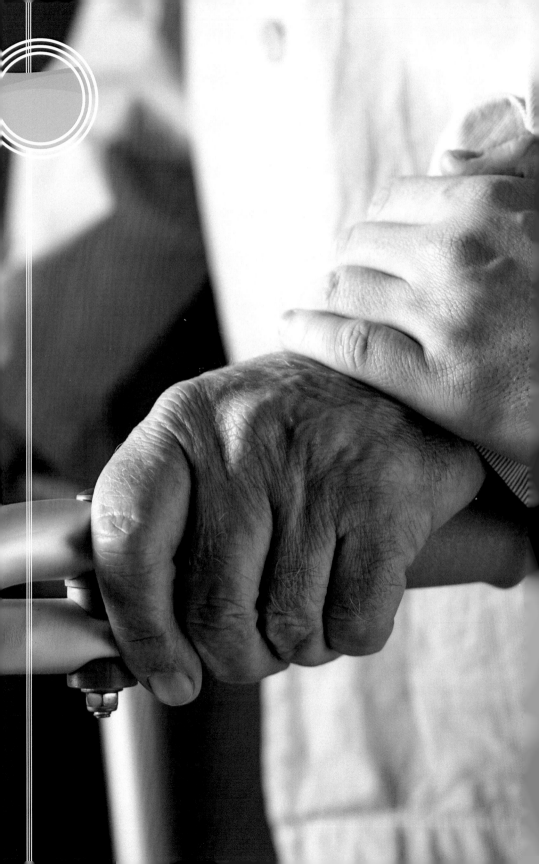

FRANCIS

NEW WAYS TO BE WITH MY DAD

FRANCIS IS MARRIED AND HAS THREE GROWN SONS. HE LIVES IN Upstate New York and is a professor of psychology, education, and human services in New York's state university system. In addition to maintaining a counseling practice, he presents seminars and workshops around the country on various aspects of midlife transition.

That's the kind of information you'll find in his résumé. But Francis would rather talk about his dad and his experience as a caregiver. Being a caregiver during the last years of his father's life brought about many personal realizations for Francis. "My relationship with my dad in those years of his illness fed my own midlife growing experience," he told me. Here's his caregiver story.

My father lived in the family home my grandfather had built, which he was very attached to. I helped him maintain his independence and live there as long as he was able to. My dad was always self-sufficient, but when he became ill he needed help, and I took on the role of caregiver.

I wanted everything in my father's care to be perfect. I was determined to be the perfect caregiver. Eventually I saw that there were many things connected with his illness that I had no control over, but at that time I thought if I handled it all perfectly, I could make him well. I was going to do everything right and keep him alive another ten or more years. I was so busy making things right that I didn't acknowledge reality. The truth was that he knew he was going to die.

For months, I was involved in *doing*. I had to constantly be doing something for my dad. I would get done working at the college, see my private clients, get to my dad's house at seven at night, make his dinner, change his bed, do the laundry, give him his medication, clean the house, get his meals ready for the next day, and leave a little after nine. I'd do that every night.

One day, I realized that I was trying to fix everything. I don't know how or when it happened, but I came to accept that my dad wasn't going to get well; that I couldn't fix him. Somehow I had touched on the wisdom that all my efforts might make him comfortable, but I couldn't make him well. Then I was ready to learn another lesson.

Every once in a while my dad would say, "Hey, Francis, why don't you sit down with me and talk?" But I'd always say, "No time for that, Dad. Sorry." I had gotten caught up in doing stuff around the house, in the routine care of my dad. Then one day I was driving home and it suddenly hit me. My dad was asking me to stop doing the "stuff" and to sit down with him, talk with him, share with him my day, and simply let him express his thoughts. He was asking me to listen to him. And when this hit me, a voice in my head said, "Hey, I'm so busy *doing* that I've got no time for *being*." I suddenly became aware that this was an opportunity that would never come again. Anyone could do the household stuff, but no one could be with my dad like I could, and no person in the world could be with me like my father.

So, things changed. I started to get other people to do the chores so that when I went over to the house I could just be with him. Sometimes we would go out to lunch and just spend time together talking. There were a lot of things I wanted to know about him and the family and to understand before he died. As we talked more and more, I felt I was touching my roots in a way I never had before. I felt like I was a little kid again.

These were our best times together. We talked about his early childhood, and I began to understand my father in a different way. My father's father, my grandfather, left Italy when my father was five, and he worked in the United States for a number of years. When my father was ten, his father brought him to the United States. After only one year his father went back to Italy, saying he'd return with the rest of the family. But he didn't, and my dad never saw him again. I began to get a deeper understanding of who my father was, how his childhood and early years had shaped him. My dad was thinking deeply about the meaning of his life, his values, the way he had conducted his business, and how proud he was of what he had accomplished. We talked about family, and I told him how much he had given me and how much our getting close in these last months meant to me. We talked about his mother, whom he hadn't seen since he was a child. He said he was dreaming about her a lot, maybe because he knew he was dying and would be seeing her soon. That's when I started to cry, and he teared up too. Italian men aren't supposed to cry, but we were both deeply touched. We had entered another level of our relationship, an intimacy we'd never had before.

Dad moved in with us for the last five months of his life. Up until that time we had done all we could to keep him in his own home. About three weeks before Dad died, I took time off from work and canceled all my speaking engagements and other appointments. Lo and behold, the world didn't end. People said, "It's okay. You need to be where you need to be." It was a real lesson in humility. You're important, but you're not that important. The world will go on while you do what you need to do.

Being busy, filling every minute with *doing*, neglects part of what people need in their lives. We never know what tomorrow is going to bring. I had heard the words for years—people talking about living in the moment—but I didn't understand; I hadn't lived it. Changing the priorities in my life gave me the chance to learn that my dad was really special. I came to understand that he was a deep thinker and a philosopher. Getting to know my father, and to know him so intimately, helped me understand more about myself. Looking back, the illness I had damned for so long had, in truth, offered me a new way to be with my dad. Without his dependency on me and my participation in his care, I might never have experienced or understood what I came to learn. I hope I never forget.

———————————————

Over many years I've talked with family caregivers about the dramatic changes required to manage the needs and schedules of their spouse, children, and job while accommodating the person in their care. Only rarely have they spoken of sharing relaxed conversation as a priority in their caregiving schedule.

Many caregivers are adult children who are married, have full-time jobs, have children of various ages, and are also committed to activities in their community, religious congregation, or other groups. Our lives have become complicated and demanding. Many adult children who take on managing the care of an ill or now limited and aging parent focus on efficiently assuming this new responsibility and challenge.

With a goal of accommodating the new and constantly changing needs of a parent or relative, efficiency and planning is necessary. Rarely does abundant time remain for an often unexpressed need of the person in care—deep personal conversation. Of course, each situation is different, yet each is governed by a new need fitting into an already often overloaded and demanding schedule. The obvious external caregiving responsibilities are taken on, yet that often creates other unspoken needs.

Persons in care find that as contacts with friends diminish and activities become fewer, they feel more isolated. From an outsider point of view we can see clearly the needs and pressures of the family caregiver. We can also empathize with the needs and desires of the one in care. Days unexpectedly become empty, lonely, and totally different from the established pattern of a person's life. A change in one's ability to engage in physical activities, a diagnosis of a disease or an injury, a loss of a wife, husband, or life partner, or other changes or challenges now require the assistance of a relative. That relative, often a grown-up, married child, now has only the time for practical things, necessities such as taking the parent to a doctor appointment, preparing meals for the next day so the parent will eat, doing the laundry, the shopping, and other chores. No time for a positive answer to a request such as "Hey, can you sit down and talk with me?"

1. How can you as a family caregiver change a situation so that the sociability needs of the person in care are recognized? How can you create an atmosphere other than "You need this done, and it's my job to do it!"?

2. How can you establish a partnership between yourself as

caregiver and the person now in care? How would you need to redefine your caregiver role?

3. Where in your community could (or do) family caregivers meet and talk about things that aren't working well in their particular caregiving situation?

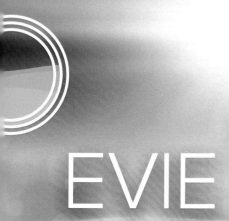

EVIE

PARTNERS IN CAREGIVING

BILL HAS MULTIPLE SCLEROSIS. AT THE TIME OF OUR CONVER-
sations, Bill's wife, Evie, was sixty-eight and Bill was seventy-nine.
For many couples, retirement is a time to travel and explore new
things. Yet, for some couples, illness and other limitations prevent
pursuing such adventures. Recently Evie and Bill moved from
their Northern California retirement community to Colorado to live
closer to their adult children. The decision was difficult, yet everyone realized that Evie and Bill needed their family's help and support. I've known Evie and Bill for many years, so I was comfortable
taking my tape recorder along on a visit and asking Evie to talk
about her caregiving experience. Here's what she told me.

Where should I begin? My husband, Bill, has multiple sclerosis. When I married him I knew he had multiple sclerosis, but I had no idea what I was getting into. It was the second marriage for both of us. People warned us about the possibilities of total disability, but it was too late—we were madly in love. Bill was diagnosed with MS in 1980. We were married in 1984. He was still walking then but with a bit of an uneven gait. He soon began using a cane, then a walker, a scooter, and later, a wheelchair. When Bill first began using a wheelchair, he could operate it himself. Over the years he's lost the use of his hands, so he has to be fed, bathed, and transferred in and out of bed. We have an automobile that has a conversion for the wheelchair, so we're able to get around. I'm strong enough to load and unload Bill and the wheelchair wherever we go. It's our lifeline, our access to the world. We decided a long time ago that we were going to use some of our savings to make our lives easier. The van was expensive, and I remember thinking we should be saving money for that "rainy day," and Bill said, "Maybe this is it."

I've been a caregiver in some measure all these years. My life is totally organized around Bill's care. As his disease changes and alters his needs, my caregiving responsibilities change too. Bill is considered a quadriplegic. We have an aide who comes in three mornings a week, gives him a shower and a shave, and does some physical therapy with him. The other four days a week I get him out of bed, give him a shower, transferring him with a patient lift to a shower chair and back to bed to dress him. I am here for all our meals and feed Bill. A lot of days we eat only two meals; we don't have a set routine. I brush his teeth, change his catheter, read to him, order books for him to listen to, take him to movies, try to visit friends if their homes are accessible, and on and on. Thankfully, he has a bright mind and no cognitive impairment.

Just to give you an idea of some of our expenses, the aide is thirty dollars an hour. On the mornings the aide is here, I'm able to leave for a couple of hours and take the dog for a run. Then I come back and get ready for the day. The thing that has changed most, and I don't remember quite when this happened, is that I can't leave Bill alone, so I'm able to get away for short periods on my own only if someone comes to be with him. The hardest part for me as a caregiver is not having the ease of spontaneously getting away. One challenge is finding the right person to stay here when I leave, and the other concern is the cost.

The truth is that I really don't enjoy being away from Bill. I much prefer to take him with me, but that's not always possible, because not every place I want to go is accessible to him. We do have an extraordinary relationship. It's very open, and we're able to resolve issues. Yes, Bill is dependent, but we need to make decisions together to have our relationship work.

People sometimes ask who takes care of me. This caregiver takes care of the caregiver! That's very, very important. It's right up there with taking care of Bill. I take good care of myself, and I keep busy. I do some hiking, exercising, yoga, grocery shopping—anything that helps me get some time on my own and keep a positive attitude so I can carry on my caregiving responsibilities. And I get a lot of support from Bill. He encourages me to take care of myself, to work out, to take time to do for myself what I need to do. I work some too out of my home office. I'm the resource editor for the National Family Caregivers Association. I review books, tapes, products, and services and write the resource page for our newsletter. It helps me keep informed and helps others. Occasionally I'm asked to speak or do a workshop, and sometimes Bill and I do a presentation together for local groups.

One positive aspect of my caregiving is that I feel useful, important. It's a very good feeling to have an opportunity right here in my own house to make a difference, and that's rewarding. At times, of course, others need to help me—when there's a medical problem or something complex that I can't understand. I enjoy trying to figure some things out for myself, though. Sometimes when something in our house isn't working properly or a piece of Bill's equipment is broken, Bill says, "Call somebody," and I'll say, "No wait. Let me see if I can figure it out first." I like to figure out how to fix something, how to solve a problem, how to make whatever Bill needs work better for him. That helps me feel needed, useful, and competent.

I do have times when I get frustrated and irritated. But that doesn't have to do with Bill. It's when equipment breaks down or repair people don't show up or we've hired somebody and they can't do what they said they could—that kind of thing. My frustrating, irritating, dark times are usually connected with equipment not working, how much money it takes for the care Bill needs, or how hard it is to find and keep competent help. Then there's the continuing difficulty of dealing with the health-care system. When I get sick (although that doesn't happen very often) or when Bill gets sick, sometimes I just lose it. I get scared that I can't handle it, and sometimes I scream and yell and say nasty, mean things. I remember once I screamed, "Maybe you should be in a nursing home," which, of course, I didn't really mean. It doesn't happen often, but when I act out like this, Bill just gets very quiet, closes his eyes, and lets me rant and rave. And then I feel totally drained, and the episode is over and I'm okay again.

Last October Bill was rushed to the hospital with what we thought was a stroke but turned out to be a raging bladder infection that had to be watched carefully. When people with MS get any infection, their whole system shuts down. The scene in the emergency room was frightening and frustrating for me. I was trying to be calm, but it was difficult for me not knowing if Bill was going to be okay. They wanted to give him a broad-spectrum antibiotic and other treatments, but before I'd agree to anything I wanted an explanation and more information. The medical personnel wanted me to leave the room, but I wouldn't go. I was exhausted and furious.

I finally got through to them, but if I hadn't been persistent, aggressive, and informed, it wouldn't have happened. They simply do not understand the role of the family caregiver. Our coverage entitled Bill to home health care after being released from the hospital. They sent over nursing help that was inept and totally inexperienced with someone in Bill's condition. I could hardly stand it. I could yell and scream all I wanted, but that was the only person who was available and that's why they sent her. It's situations like this that get me down. The health-care system is a source of great frustration to us much of the time.

People ask how I do it. I don't think of it like that. We do it one day at a time. What's changed over the years is that we've had increasing limitations, so we've had to supplement or sublimate or—I don't know what the correct word would be—maybe just substitute. We manage to find ways to entertain ourselves and do some of the things we still enjoy, while letting go of the other things. I look at my life as a caregiver in a positive way. Most of the time it is, about eighty-twenty. I think Bill, who's the care recipient, feels the same way. About

80 percent of the time he sees his life in a positive way, and then 20 percent of the time there are other feelings of loss and negativity. That would be a good enough balance for any of us in life.

I find caregiving for Bill challenging but extraordinarily gratifying. I know I'm making a difference in his life, and that's where my gratification comes from. I feel so much joy while watching him get pleasure out of what we're doing together. My caregiving isn't a frustrating task for me, because it gives me a great deal back. I think it's because of the person I'm giving the care to.

Bill is an extraordinary guy. He's always willing to learn. He's a lot of fun. He has an open, inquisitive mind, and that gives me a lot. He's an inspiration for me. There's great love and affection here. I truly feel like we're doing this together. I don't feel alone. Bill gives me tremendous affirmation as a woman, a wife, a mother, and a grandmother. He's very affirming of everything I do for him and with him. He exudes love for me, constantly telling me how wonderful I am. One night we went to a concert, and during intermission a man we didn't know came over and said to me, "I've been watching you and your husband. It touches my heart to see so much love. Your affection for each other truly shows." That he would come over to us and say such things really amazed me. If people have some purpose in this world, maybe this is ours: to show people what true love looks like.

I'm learning that I can be patient. Deeper rewards, spiritual rewards have also come to me as a caregiver. Millions of people in our world need help. I have only one person to help, but, in a way, I feel like I'm helping the whole world. It feels good inside to help someone else, whether by giving a hand to someone who is homeless or even by sending money to cancer research. I'm fortunate enough to be reminded of it every minute of every day.

Sometimes I say to myself, "What would I be doing with my life if I wasn't doing this?" I don't feel deprived. People are always telling me they admire me. People I don't even know come up to me and say that. Actually, what I do isn't that hard. It's time consuming, sure, but this is my life, after all. I don't want people to misunderstand and think this is easy. It's not easy; but it is doable.

The biggest reward of caregiving for me is finding out what's really important in life and focusing on that. I'm not preoccupied by or encumbered with possessions. It's more important for us just to share our lives together than to have material things. When I'm out with other people and they're dressed nicer than I am or they look more put together, I'm okay with that. I know who I am, and I found this out through caregiving. I know where my priorities are, what my values are. I feel so good that I don't need those other things. That's my reward.

There's an intimacy about caregiving that I enjoy. Our giving and taking has mutuality; we're partners in caregiving. I don't think this is always the way it is between caregiver and the people being cared for.

From time to time I'll see couples walking arm in arm and wonder what that would feel like. But then I also see people dealing with heart disease, cancer, hearing loss, vision loss, and any number of ailments and ills, and I wonder what that would be like. Would I be able to deal with that? Recently I read a sentence that really spoke to me: "I live the life that is before me." That's it. That's what I do. What I've gained through caregiving is a deep and profound understanding of compassion—compassion, not just for the person I care for, but for everyone who needs caregiving, for everyone who gives care. It's my deepest learning, my greatest gift.

———————————————

Most often we hear about caregiver situations in a marriage that develop after a couple has been together a number of years. Evie and Bill went into their marriage aware of the reality that Bill had been diagnosed with multiple sclerosis. However, they didn't know how slowly or quickly deterioration might come. Bill needed some care, although minimal, in the early months of their marriage. Evie told me that for her, caring for Bill's health was part of their marriage arrangement. "I feel like we're doing this together," she said.

I had never heard a family caregiver describe their caregiving relationship as Evie did when she referred to her caregiving for Bill as a partnership. But I'm beginning to see that attitude emerge in a few couples I know socially. This perspective actually influenced both my attitude and my actions in my recent care for my husband as he lived his final years. "We" made both large and small decisions together. Our days began by deciding together if it was a day he needed help to put on his socks or he felt he could try to do it alone.

I'm also seeing an attitude of partnership in the management of some long-term care situations, nursing homes, and other living arrangements for people requiring various levels of care. I've observed a trend toward deliberately cultivating friendship between the person who performs the caregiving and the person in care. Of course, needs related to physical assistance and prescribed medical care continue to be primary and necessary concerns in the relationship. Some small care homes for eight to ten people and a few larger units are reflecting less of an institutional attitude. The professional nurse, social worker, or other people working with clients are competent and sensitive. Yet, the feeling that "because you're the patient in my care, I'm the person in charge of all decisions" is less evident.

I believe that in any caregiving situation, whether it's in a professional care residence or in a family home, offering a warm word, holding a hand, or exchanging a smile is a welcome gift to a person in care. Such gestures of caring and friendship lighten a stressful atmosphere. Sometimes the dirty dishes in the sink, the unfolded laundry, or the bed linen that could be changed can wait while a family caregiver shares a cup of tea or fifteen minutes just sitting in the garden with the loved one in care.

1. **What stories in your work or personal caregiving situation can you share about persons neglecting to take time for themselves, becoming ill and worn out in their commitment to caregiving for another? What stories can you tell of caregivers who realized the truth in the words, "You need to take care of yourself so you can take care of another"?**

2. **What situations are you aware of in which the nature of the relationship between caregivers and those receiving care has been changed, by policy and training, to encourage partnership?**

3. **What are your observations about the relationships between caregivers and those in care?**

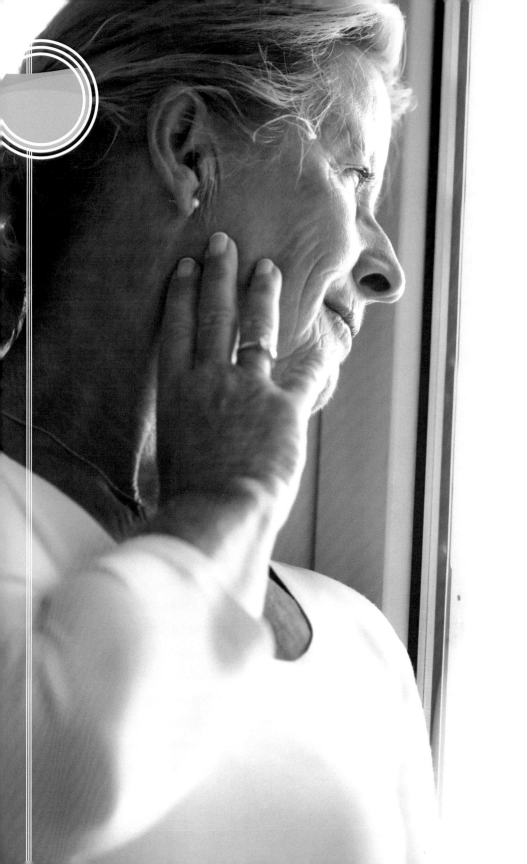

SHARON

I WOULDN'T TRADE THOSE YEARS

SHARON IS FIFTY-EIGHT YEARS OLD. SHE LIVES ALONE IN A SPA-
cious, charming old home, surrounded by antique furniture and
mementos of a life with her partner, Sheila, who passed away
three years earlier. We sat comfortably in her fragrant and colorful
backyard garden, sipping our iced tea as Sharon told me about
Sheila and their life together.

Before we met, Sheila had been married and had four
children. I've known her children for many years
now, and they consider me like a second mom. When
Sheila's father died and she was helping her mother clean out
his closet, Sheila's mother said to her, "You know, for over fifty
years I was married to your dad, and I never really felt like
I was loved." And Sheila thought, "I've just put in nineteen
years unloved. I'm making a decision. I'm not going to do it
anymore!" She subsequently got a divorce.

I met Sheila when I was thirty-nine; she was seven years
older than me. We'd be together almost seventeen years. After
Sheila and I moved in together, one of our friends said that

seeing the two of us leave for work gave her quite a laugh. Two lawyers going to work—Sheila with her little Peter Pan collar, pearls, and proper business suit. And then me in my hippie sandals, peasant skirt, and cloth briefcase.

Sheila had been a stay-at-home mom, but she was exceptionally smart. While in her forties she took the required tests, got into law school, and eventually became the county law librarian. All the judges, lawyers, and law clerks loved her. When you were in a conversation with her you knew she was really interested in you, and she was always doing things for everyone she knew. Sheila was a very special, unique person. She loved people, and when you were in her presence you always felt really special—everybody did.

When Sheila started getting sick, the only symptom she had was an uncharacteristic depression. Then she started doing odd things. Like one day a friend slammed her car door shut while Sheila's finger was in the door. She never said a word, just pulled it out. She didn't cry out or say anything, but her finger was broken. Then she started having dizzy spells and fell a couple of times at work. The care the doctors suggested didn't help. She got worse every day. We finally went to the Mayo Clinic, and they found brain tumors. They did brain surgery and discovered that she had central nervous system lymphoma. It's rare. Only about 2 percent of the population gets this form of cancer. We had some big decisions to make. We decided we didn't want to be away from each other, so I closed my law office, said good-bye to my secretary and my paralegal, and stayed at home to be with Sheila for the time we had left together.

"I think I have this illness for a reason," Sheila told me. When I asked her to elaborate, she explained that she felt that having this disease was to teach people something important, to teach people about living and cancer. She asked that we make a conscious decision to deal with her illness and share a positive perspective. So, we made a pact that we weren't going to get angry about little stuff, because we didn't want to use our energy that way. We immediately saw so many things in our lives that were small compared to what we were faced with now.

During the months that followed I learned a lot about grace. I watched Sheila deal with things in an amazing way, things that for me would have been insurmountable. She had full brain radiation and chemotherapy. After the treatments she would always thank the nurses. She was never cross or irritable. She didn't complain, not once. I never heard her say, "Why is this happening to me?" or "Why do I have to go through this?" As I watched her I learned something very important about how to look at what comes to us during our lives. I began to see that questioning what you've been given isn't of any value, because it keeps you stuck in the same place, and actually looking backward. Through Sheila's example I learned that when you're given something, that's what it is. The challenge is to find the best and most beneficial meaning out of that experience.

Over time Sheila became more and more childlike. Somehow I was able to learn to accept and balance both the adult and the child in her. I couldn't have the same kind of conversations with her as I'd had in the past, but I realized that we just had to let our relationship shift. I took Sheila out for lunch every day so she would have some life out in the world, and I learned to put her needs and her moods before mine. I'm sure it was the tumor that caused her to say inappropriate, crazy things out of context. Like one day when we were on an escalator and she yelled out, "Don't push me off!" or we'd be at a friend's home talking and having tea, and she'd say, "Don't run over me with the car, Sherry." My challenge was to learn to live with things like this and not take what she blurted out that seriously.

Sheila lived five and a half years after she was diagnosed, but she was quite compromised after the surgery. Spending all the time I could with Sheila in those remaining years of her life was important to me. We developed a new kind of intimacy, a different kind of closeness because she became so childlike. I felt it was inappropriate to have an adult physical intimacy with her, but we hugged and sat close and held hands. It was hard for me to leave her side even to take care of the dog, go shopping, or do the laundry. She always wanted me to be in the same room with her. One day when I was out of the room for just minutes, she called out rather desperately, "Sherry, come in here now and be with me. I'm so lonesome!" During the last months of her life I moved my computer right next to her bed so I could be there all the time.

I remember several things Sheila said to me toward the end. One day, out of nowhere, she said, "You know, Sherry, it's always easier to be kind." I now try always to be considerate and understanding. I so often think how Sheila might react in a situation, and her words "Be kind" echo in my head. I've become more compassionate and sensitive to the mood and frame of mind of others.

I've learned other things from my caregiving experience. Martyring ourselves because we have to take care of another person doesn't help the situation at all. I want to caution people who are caring for a loved one to watch out for that. I used to ask myself, "Am I doing enough? Is there more I should do to make Sheila happy and comfortable? Am I spending enough time with her?" I know now that it accomplishes nothing to agonize about such things. I know too that many of us struggle with feelings that we should always do more and more. You do what you can and accept that.

Another thing: I was wrong not to let others help me. So many of our friends offered, but I'd say no. I was determined to do it all myself. They finally stopped asking and would just show up with a meal or ice cream or insist on staying with Sheila while I went out. For some of us it's hard to accept help. Yet, a person can't show that they're truly your friend unless you let them in and allow them to help. They want to be part of the caregiving process, and you deprive them of that if you don't allow them to participate.

I wouldn't trade those years I took care of Sheila for anything. I never made the house like a sick place. I always had colorful sheets on Sheila's hospital bed, flowers in the room, and tea and cookies when friends stopped over. For me, caring for Sheila was a joyful, marvelous thing. I never saw it as a hardship or a burden; I felt it was a wonderful journey and that I was privileged to be a part of it. I felt like I was giving back in some way the many years of giving and companionship that Sheila had given to me.

In my conversation with Sharon there was an atmosphere of quiet calm as she spoke of her late partner, Sheila, and told me of the many things she had learned from her during the time she provided care for her partner. When Sharon reflected on her caregiving experience she realized that her refusal of help from friends was a mistake. She understood only after Sheila died that her constant refusal of the offers from friends deprived them of participating in the care of their close friend Sheila. Her competence and determination to control every aspect of her partner's care deprived others of the chance to be involved in the care of their friend. In Sharon's admission of her mistake about this, her new awareness of her need to assume control might be a learning she can bring to other areas of her life.

1. Tell a story about a caregiver who felt the need to take control of everything for the person requiring the care, the household, and other needs but learned to let others participate. If you haven't had such an experience, how might you deal with the desire to control in the future?

2. What thoughts and feelings did you have about Sharon's description of the childlike behavior that evolved as Sheila's condition deteriorated? If you have ever dealt with such a situation, share your story with others to help them grow in their awareness of the experience.

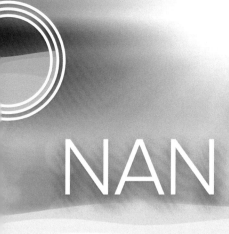

NAN

ONE BIG LESSON

I ARRIVED AT NAN'S SUBURBAN HOME JUST IN TIME FOR OUR appointment. I didn't know her, hadn't even spoken with her on the telephone. A mutual friend had made the contact, and the message I received was that Nan was eager to talk with me. At that time I was scheduling conversations with parents who were caregivers for children with special needs. I was delighted for the opportunity to speak with her and most appreciative that she was so willing to talk with me. Nan was generous, not only with her hospitality, but also in sharing with me, and with you, her heartfelt and deeply touching story.

As you begin to read Nan's story you may think, "This story has nothing to do with my life. Maybe I'll skip it and go on to the next." But I encourage you to keep reading.

Being a caregiver is the way I define myself and my life, for better or for worse, no matter what other roles I play. I am a psychotherapist, which is work I love, and I'm a wife, a friend, a daughter, and a sister. But what really defines almost every moment for me is being a mom. My older son, Jason—we call him Jay—is seventeen; my younger son, Aaron, is fourteen. Both boys have cerebral palsy. Our older son is severely disabled. He uses a wheelchair and doesn't have the use of his hands. Although Jay's speech has been affected, we can understand him most of the time. There was a time when we thought he wouldn't talk at all. Now he speaks nonstop. He is delightful and sweet and funny. My youngest son is mildly affected. He uses crutches and has impairments, but they are not as limiting as my older son.

Cerebral palsy is an umbrella description for a group of disorders related to muscle and movement control, visual disorders, seizures, and various sensory disabilities believed to originate in the brain. There's not one specific cause of cerebral palsy. At one time it was believed cerebral palsy resulted from injury to the brain before, during, or immediately after birth. New theories suggest other possible causes, such as abnormal brain development, insufficient circulation to areas of the brain, an infection in the brain, or bleeding in the brain. Whatever the cause, this is what we live with.

Jay was born two months premature, but we were told he was fine. It was the end of October. The weather was very cold, and I was told to keep him in. He cried constantly. I was a new mom, and I felt inadequate to parent a child who was so miserable. The baby would cry, and then I would cry. I couldn't soothe him, and everyone was giving me advice. A friend of mine had a child at about the same time, and her perfect little baby never cried. To be unable to comfort my child was not a good feeling. If there had been a diagnosis, it would have been easier. But it was nine months before the doctor finally told us that Jay had cerebral palsy.

With no family history of cerebral palsy, we dared to get pregnant again. It was devastating to find out Aaron also had cerebral palsy. Thankfully, he was not as severely affected. I dived headfirst into the care of the boys, even though I was depressed and had so much to do and adjust to. It's gotten easier as the boys have gotten older. The demands are different, and I've discovered more about how to take care of myself. I know that's the bottom line for any caregiver: to take care of yourself so you can care for others. It's hard to remember that.

Something I've learned along the way is not to judge the choices other people make. That is a hard thing to do. We're all raised in some ways to be judgmental, but I've learned now not to judge anyone else's choices. For example, so many people ask me why I didn't put my boys in an institution. Some people might make that choice; it might be right for them. But it never occurred to us to do anything but have them at home.

I'm well aware that some marriages fall apart under the stress of having children with special needs. Our marriage has, thankfully, survived the strain. Through the years, we've grown into our individual roles, though it hasn't been easy. My husband and I are able to talk now about how, at one time, he wished he could escape. And I can tell him about the many times I've wanted to run away too. We've sheltered each other. He'd drive by a park and see some father throwing a ball to his son, and it would hurt, but he wouldn't tell me how miserable that made him feel, because he didn't want to hurt me more. And I did the same. I'd keep quiet about my feelings. For a while I resented my husband for not being more involved. Now I've learned to ask him for help in a way he can hear. It's been uneven for us. We haven't always been able to be mutually supportive.

We're fortunate to have loving and supportive families. Both sets of grandparents have been phenomenal. My husband's parents have embraced the boys and have been an amazing part of their lives. And one of my father's great joys was spending time with the boys too. I have a photo album of him with the boys, and they are laughing in all the pictures. You never knew he was dealing with children with special needs. Some families aren't there for them. We are very blessed.

You cannot be down around these kids, because they aren't. They are so upbeat. The older one always has pain, and yet he doesn't complain. Jay will say, "My head itches" or "My eye itches." I am constantly struck by what it must be like not to be able to rub your eye. I am always faced with what these children can't do, the many things we take for granted. It helps me be patient with them, even though it puts constant demands on me. Yet, no matter how lousy my day has been, when I look at these children at the end of the day, I can't help but put all my little stuff in a petty category and embrace a healthy life perspective, and live one day at a time.

Neither one of the boys defines himself as disabled, which is fascinating to us. They are aware of their disabilities, but that is not their first definition of themselves. One day we were visiting a radio station and hanging out with the disc jockey. It was great fun. About a week later Aaron called up to request a song and said, "Hi, we were there a few weeks ago." And he went on to describe his hair color and other things that would identify him, but he never said they were the kids with the wheelchair and the walker. That's not how he describes himself or his brother.

One day I was driving Jason to a recreation program, and he yakked so much I could hardly concentrate on driving. We pulled up, and I was thinking that I desperately needed some quiet time. In the car next to us was a boy wearing an oxygen mask. I thought, "Thank you, God. Thank you for that reminder." Life has handed me a number of these experiences. I took Aaron to a therapist one day, and I was sitting in the waiting room next to the receptionist. As the receptionist tried to schedule an appointment with another client, I heard the client say, "No, I can't come that day. That's the day I have my chemotherapy." Again, "Thank you, God."

Because of my children, I have grown enormously. But this is not growth anyone would go looking for. This is not something you choose. The growth has been painful and difficult, and yet it has given me amazing perspective on life. That I'll be caregiving for my entire life is scary to contemplate. Knowing this has made me more conscious of my health. I owe it to my children to be as healthy as I can be. We don't know what the future holds. Yet we know that in our lifetime we will always be caregivers.

It is easier seventeen years later, but there are moments and situations arising all the time that are difficult. It's still one day at a time. It's a life lesson. How else is there to really live? None of us knows what will be.

Caregivers need to feel free and comfortable to express their feelings. You need to find someone to whom you can say, "At this moment, I hate this. I hate my kid. I hate my husband." You don't want to stay stuck there, but if you can't say it, you are in big trouble. You need to complain. You can't stuff the feelings. You need a support system. You need to say things you thought you couldn't imagine yourself saying. Call a friend. You've got to be heard, and you've got to be open with your feelings. If you can't find a way to share those most awful feelings, you cannot go on.

We are all tempted to look at another person's situation with envy. We're jealous of those who seem to have more or have it easier. But someone is always richer, luckier, or healthier. We can spend our lives being bitter, or we can look at our own lives with different eyes and see how blessed we are. What is really important? What really matters? I can look outside myself. I can have a larger view of life.

People often say to us, "We couldn't do what you do." The truth is you do what you have to. There's that line I've gotten so tired of hearing: "God never gives you anything you can't handle." I don't want to be in a position to know how much harder it could be. This feels like enough, thank you very much. We don't always get to choose what we get in life. And that's a big thing for me, recognizing what we can choose and what we can't choose. Being angry and bitter isn't useful for anybody. I can say to others that no matter what, you can live through it and you will. And I live that myself, one day at a time. That's the one big lesson.

There was an aura of peace and serenity in the room as Nan told me the story of her two sons. I believe Nan's story is about each of us, though not in the specifics of her particular situation but in how we deal with the complicated challenges that may come into our own lives.

Nan and her husband have faced sadness, anger, struggles, and disappointment. Both admitted that many times each wanted to run away and leave a situation that couldn't be fixed. Reading their story may suggest ways of understanding and accepting our own often challenging situations, which can also elicit complicated feelings and responses. Once again we are reminded that we can learn and grow from a story very different from our own.

Possibly Nan's profession as a psychotherapist has given her skills for adapting to situations that can't be changed yet involve every member of a family. Maybe that was also a factor in her acceptance of their sons' disabilities. Possibly her professional training influenced the forming of her sons' self-images in positive ways. However, Nan's story supports my belief that each of us is able to move disappointment, anger, and bitterness out of our way. Nan's perspective is we begin doing that by being honest about both the good and the bad feelings regarding our situation and by deciding to live one day at a time. Maybe her comment about what she described as a particularly lousy day are her gift to us. "When I look at these children at the end of the day, I can't help but put all my little stuff in a petty category and embrace a healthy life perspective, and live one day at a time."

1. What challenges or situations similar to Nan and her husband's are you or your clients dealing with? What has it been like for you to address such extreme family challenges in either your personal or your work life?

2. What suggestions can you offer people trying to cope with temporary breakdowns or emotional upheavals? How can a person learn to forgive him- or herself in such situations?

3. What other thoughts has Nan's story brought up for you? What problems, family situations, or other challenges have come into your life?

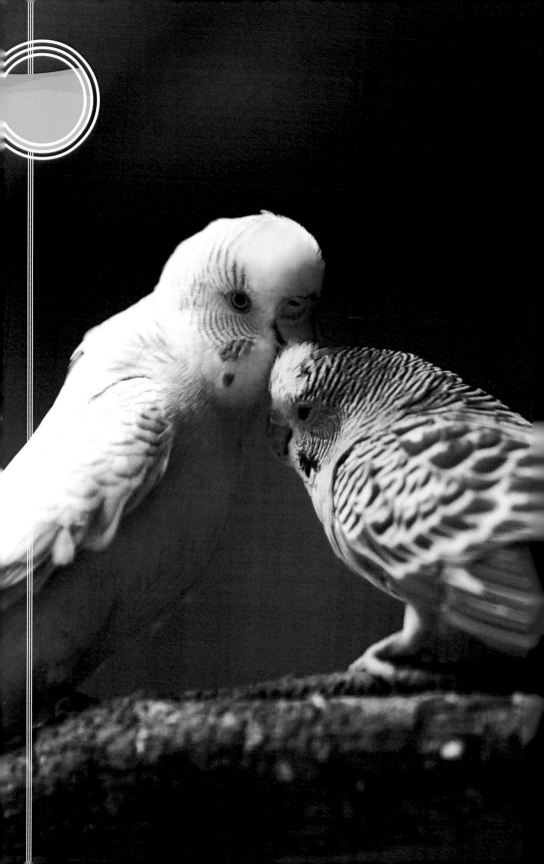

RICHARD

SPEAKING EACH OTHER'S LANGUAGES

ALTHOUGH I'VE USED ONLY FIRST NAMES IN THE MAJORITY OF the conversations shared in this book, I've included a few well-known personalities. For many, it will quickly become evident that this conversation was with the well-known and highly respected photographer Richard Avedon. I met Richard in July 1970. He was at the Minneapolis Institute of Art getting ready for what was labeled "the first showing of his serious work" following several years of success in fashion photography. I was a middle-aged student in graduate school at the University of Minnesota, working part time at the campus radio station as the arts reporter. Our friendship continued until his death in 2004.

I remember arriving at the museum as he was preparing to take a break from hanging his exhibition. A dozen reporters had waited patiently for an interview but were eventually told there would be no possibility for questions. Most of the reporters left. Being persistent and determined, I followed Richard into the park across from the museum where he was sitting under a tree. I approached him with a request for a brief conversation, and when he surprised me by saying yes, I turned on my tape recorder, and we began discussing the obvious subject, his photography. Our conversation took an unexpected turn, and I found myself listening to the poignant and personal story of his relationship with his father.

Over the last years of his father's life Richard took an extensive series of photos of him. The portraits chronicle his father as he changed from an alert, well-dressed man in his eighties into a withered victim of terminal cancer. He told me that a question often put to him about this series of photographs was "What kind of a son would take pictures of his dying father?" Richard responded that the photos represented not only his father, or what he felt for his father, but anyone at the end of life.

Some of the conversation you'll read here was originally heard as a public radio broadcast in 1970. Several years later I had another opportunity to interview Richard when an exhibition of his more recent photographs was on view in Washington, DC. Some of that conversation is also included here.

We weren't very close as father and son, actually not close at all. When I was young, he was a schoolteacher and had a very tough life. I think he felt that he could give me the kind of education that would strengthen me for a world he saw as a battle. But the nature of his intelligence simply wasn't the nature of mine. I was born with a visual intelligence. The pressures to learn from him, his way, were too strong, and I never had a sense I would reach the end of his demands. If I would only concentrate, he would tell me, then I could learn. Whatever he was good at, I was not; whatever he was interested in, I wasn't, and what I was interested in, he had no way of understanding. I slipped into my area of interest, photography, an interest that lasted my entire life. As far as my father was concerned, we had little to say to one another.

When he was in his sixties his marriage to my mother broke up, and he moved to Florida. Over the years, as my son grew up, I had this vivid realization that there was this stranger, living in Florida, who was my father and my son's grandfather.

It was a very conscious effort that brought me to Sarasota, Florida, to understand who my father was. It had nothing to do with my profession of photography. It was to know him and to feel that there could be something between us. I have a strong sense that life isn't meaningless and that we have to make whatever small meaning is possible out of the time we're here. I felt that if I never learned to love my father, I was betraying a possibility in life and an opportunity to pass something on to my own son. I have a great sense of continuity.

My father was retired. Then in his late seventies, he complained about everything, particularly about real estate values. At one point I had one of those great strokes of insight that come to us every once in a while. I said, "Listen, Dad. You sit here on the porch talking about real estate values. You know about these things. I have some money. Why don't we go into business together?" It was perfect. For the first time in our lives we met. I was in my forties and was interested in what he knew. So, there were phone calls in the middle of the night—"marinas are hot"—and everything in him came alive. The conversations were fascinating. And I really did learn a great deal from him. We finally had something to talk about.

At a certain point in the euphoria, I realized that it's always the same story: he's the father, I'm the son, yet he knows nothing about me. In my need to know him better, I was hyping up an interest in real estate that I really didn't have. I knew it would never work unless we were equals. I wrote to him—and it's the only letter of mine he ever kept. The letter said, "I've learned your business, and now I'm going to ask you to learn mine. Photography means to me what real estate means to you, and I hate giving the best that's in me to strangers and nothing to you."

The next time I came down to Florida, I brought an eight-by-ten camera, an assistant, a writer, and a tape recorder so he'd know I was serious. And every time I visited we had a photographic sitting. He learned what I wanted, and he was involved to the degree that he wanted to give me what I wanted. Finally we did speak each other's languages.

He has asked several times to see the pictures. I don't want to show them to him, because I don't think he'll like them. Whenever he poses for me, he smiles and becomes benign, gentle, and somehow wise. He would be very happy to see that picture of himself. But my photographs also show his impatience. I love that quality in him, but seeing it would frighten him. He isn't interested in the fact that he looks his age, eighty-three, and is still fantastically vibrant and angry, hungry for life and being alive. He's much more interested in looking sage. So, my sense of what's beautiful is very different from his.

The next three paragraphs are my adaptation from Avedon's introduction to the catalog for his 1970 exhibition at the Minneapolis Institute of Arts.

Eight months before he died, my father had a major liver operation that he had absolutely no expectation of surviving. I wheeled him into the operating room, and he had a little sedation. This man, who had never heard of Beckett, who didn't know what the word *existential* meant, looked up at me and said, "Dick, is, is; isn't, isn't." These might have been his last words if he had died.

Later, when he was on chemotherapy, I flew to Sarasota. We

had a really good week together. I smuggled him out of the hospital. I told him, "You don't have to die in the hospital. We can go out and have a good time." He began to get an idea of what my sense of humor was like. We went all over. I showed him my life. I took him to Miami, and we did one more sitting. Then I went back to New York. The day I left, he stopped eating, and five days later he was dead. I believe he stayed alive to have those last photographs taken.

Now understand this: my work is not journalism and those pictures are not about the death of a man. Others have described them that way, but many of them were done when he was in perfect health. They're about a certain kind of man in the world, about his life and who he was. And then too, those photographs are really about what it means to be any one of us at the end of our lives.

Many of us grow up feeling that one or both of our parents just don't understand us. Yet how much do we really understand them? We know what we learn about them in our interaction with them as our mother or father, but do we ever feel a desire or seek an opportunity to know them as people apart from that role in our life? Richard had a unique desire to build a father-son relationship and to understand who that person he called father was. Of particular interest to me was his creative—and successful—plan to build that relationship.

In many families a close relationship with a parent isn't desired or sought after, yet the desire to grow a meaningful parent–grown-up child relationship can appear. Developing a real understanding of how to grow and nourish such a relationship probably takes patience, planning, and an understanding not only of the parent but also of one's own needs.

1. Describe a healing process you, others in your family, or the families of friends or clients have experienced with a parent. What gave rise to the desire to pursue that process and how successful has it been? If it failed, why do you think it couldn't or didn't happen?

2. What are your observations about Richard's plan and his follow-through on creating a positive and real relationship with his father?

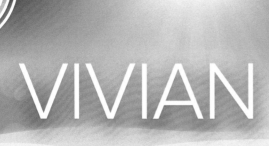

VIVIAN

A GROWING SELF-AWARENESS

VIVIAN IS A SOCIAL WORKER IN PRIVATE PRACTICE. SHE TRAVELS across the country conducting workshops and lectures on the stresses of caregiving and relationship problems between middle-aged adults and their aging parents. She didn't consider herself a writer, but after caring for each of her parents when they became ill and frail, she felt that she had important things to say. In the book she subsequently authored, she speaks of the time when we begin to notice the signs of frailty in our parents. It may be the first time we realize that they will actually grow old and die. Vivian and I shared stories about our parents' decline putting to an end whatever fantasies of their immortality we might have had. She told me, "I'm aware I had some irrational feeling that as long as my parents were alive I was protected from death. Being called upon to care for them in their declining years taught me realities about life and death, my limitations and my choices. I learned, and not easily, the things that make the difference between caregiving as a stress and caregiving as a satisfaction and a joy." I found Vivian to be a warm, compassionate, and generous conversationalist. She had gained maturity and developed wisdom from her caregiving experience.

I remember thinking that maybe I could write a book. I recall asking myself, "What do I know best?" And the answer was caregiving. I had much to say to those who are or have been caregivers for a parent. I know the hardships of caregiving, the possibilities of anger and resentment, yet I also know the rewards. I decided to use my clinical work and my personal experience to write my book, entitled *Respecting Your Limits When Caring for Aging Parents.* I knew it couldn't be just intellectual and academic or it wouldn't truly reach the reader. It had to come from my heart.

My mother was a great cook, and she loved to prepare lovely lunches for me. Although I was an adult in my middle years when I came to visit my mother, I'd again become the little girl feasting on all her delights! One day I came in and the table wasn't set. Mom said, "I haven't been able to set the table, will you help me? And maybe you could make the tuna salad. And would you wash the lettuce?" From that day on I realized that things would never be the same. I couldn't pretend, even when Mom invited me to lunch, that I was a little girl anymore. I think that it's when our parents get old that we begin to recognize our own mortality.

When my mother was diagnosed with Parkinson's disease, it was the beginning of my becoming a primary caregiver. In the lexicon of gerontology, I was what is called a distant caregiver, as I lived about thirty-five miles away. For quite a while, my father was wonderful in helping Mom with her care. My mother and I had our own areas of interaction, partly because it was easier for her to tell me personal things about toileting and other functions that she felt private about.

However, like some mothers and daughters, my mother and I had our difficulties. My mother was a very reserved person, and I tended to be quite outspoken in comparison. At times I really don't think she liked me much. She would always compare me to soft-spoken girls. I felt that I was never quite good enough for my mother. I played the piano, but my mother would tell me that my cousin played the piano better. I did well in school, but I didn't measure up in her eyes because another cousin was Phi Beta Kappa. That friction was always there.

But when I became her caregiver something wonderful happened. She thanked me many times for taking care of her. About ten or eleven years before she died, I went back to school to get a degree in social work, and my mother was actually proud of me. She told me how wonderful it was that I was going to earn my own living and be independent. Before she died she said to me, "I could never be jealous of anyone else's daughter." It seemed so easy for her to say these things. Suddenly I was something wonderful. I had triumphed in some way.

I'm now a social worker. Before I took on the caregiver responsibility of my mother, I was on the geriatric evaluation team of a family medicine residency program. I ran a caregiver support group, and I used to see adult children who weren't taking care of their parents as I thought they should.

They would tell about their parents making what they considered unreasonable demands. They didn't want to change their lives to give what they considered an excessive amount of time to their parents. Then came the time when I took on the care of my mother.

It was a situation where my personal life and my professional life converged. Here I was running myself ragged going back and forth to attend to my mother's needs. I then remembered thinking I would be better at caregiving than they were, a more attentive and devoted child. I'm embarrassed to say that I had been pretty judgmental in those days. Well, all that changed. I began to see that in my new caregiving responsibilities I was losing all sense of boundaries. I forgot that I had a self. Everything I thought or did was about her and what I could do for her, where I could take her, how I could fulfill her every need. I didn't count; I didn't matter. I was a superwoman. I could do everything.

Eventually I came to realize how much time I was devoting to doing things for my mother, how obsessed I had become about serving her needs, and how it was taking big bites out of my life. I didn't have time or energy to do my job well, relax, read a book, play a game of tennis, go to exercise class, or even look at the newspaper. It was very unhealthy for me. I short-changed my husband too. Some of us try and try, and when we don't succeed in serving all our parents' needs, we feel more and more guilty. And then we get angry and feel terrible that we're angry, and the cycle starts all over again. I realize I got into that trap with the care of my mother.

I had to fight that urge to always be there with her for everything—not that my mother expected it of me, but I expected it of myself. I guess it was my image of what "good daughters" of that generation do. I recall a day when I had promised my mom I'd take off work and spend the day with her. I remember having a terrible migraine headache, yet I still went over to care for her. I felt obligated to serve her no matter what. Unlearning that compulsion was my biggest challenge, my most important learning in being a caregiver. I hadn't set limits. I'm sure I'm not the only caregiver who has fallen into that pattern. One lesson I eventually learned was to understand that I'm not here just to take care of my parents and that I have a life that needs attention too.

I'll also tell you about some of my other learning. Once we went to a department store, and when my mother was trying on things, I wanted to help her. Because of her Parkinson's, she couldn't button or unbutton things fast or well, and my hands were always reaching out to do the buttons, the zippers, everything. My mother chastised me. "Vivian, leave me alone!" she said loudly. "There aren't many things left that I can do by myself, but I can do my buttons. If I fumble and I'm slow, you're just going to have to be patient."

I really learned something that day, and from then on I changed the way I operated. I learned to allow for her pace, to slow myself up and learn to be comfortable and patient. I allowed plenty of time; I didn't want to be rushed. Actually, slowing down gave me the chance to savor every minute of being with her. She was tottering and frail, and I came to understand that she wanted me to just hold her arm and be with her. She wanted to know that I was there for her on her terms. It became my special time with my mother, and I felt great joy in that. I was grateful, and still am, for that insight that helped me develop patience.

The learning and new awareness I gained during my caregiving experiences were simple, yet profound. Our visits became really special; time almost stood still. We talked about many things. My mother loved to reminisce. She came to this country in 1923 and worked in the sweatshops of lower Manhattan. She had all kinds of stories to tell. She loved to talk, and I began to realize that I loved to listen. I began to know my mother better and in a different way.

As I said, one big lesson I learned from caregiving is that I'm human: I have limits and I can do only so much. I had to learn to say no when I was her caregiver. Always saying yes or "of course I'll do that" takes a toll on the caregiver. I never totally integrated this learning when I was a caregiver for my mom. However, my father outlived my mother, and during the last four years of his life, I learned to say no and respect my limits. My dad would call me and ask me to leave work and take him to the bank. But instead of jumping in the car, I learned to say, "Dad, I have too much to do today. How about tomorrow?" And there would be a long pause, and he'd say, "Well, I guess that will be okay." He learned to see that I was busy, that I worked, that I had a family, and that I had other commitments. I made a lot of time for my father, but it worked best if we negotiated it. He knew I wasn't abandoning him; he was able to see my position. And I had learned that if I paid attention to my needs, I'd actually be a better caregiver.

My father lived quite independently for four years after my mother died. Then he became frail and fell. After he left the hospital, he decided to go into a nursing home. We found a very good facility, one in which the residents were free to move around and have a social life. It became a real home to my father. He was quite content, he made friends, and he created a niche for himself there. That's another thing I learned. He showed me by his example that his personal world was inside him. His life in the nursing home held meaning for him because of who he was inside. I learned that your self is your world; you can give up all your possessions and live in one room and still have the important things you need. It really is about your inner life. And my father's inner life was rich. He would talk to me about his philosophy, his life, and many of his experiences. He was very social. He loved people and could have a conversation with anyone in the nursing home. He could connect with others, and that's so important. He also seemed happy to be by himself; he liked his own company. During those last months, he shared with me feelings about his death and dying. He wasn't afraid, yet he knew he was dying. He was a sensitive and wise person.

My father died in the nursing home in my arms. He went very gently. I held him for quite a while. He was still warm, and I wanted to feel his warmth. I think because of that experience I really don't fear death. Because I was with my father at that time, I'm now even more aware of my own mortality. Knowing that death is always there at my side doesn't take away from my life, of my joy in living. I remember leaving the nursing home and thinking how thankful I was to be alive. And then I thought that I too could be here one day, and if I am, I will make the best of it as my father did. I will be alive, I will have myself, and myself will be enough. I now savor life much more with that awareness.

I'm sixty-eight now, the eldest in the family. Yes, I'm both older and wiser. My caregiving experiences with my mother and father have been part of my journey toward a growing self-awareness. What I've written in my book on being a caregiver for aging parents I'll say here once again: "To honor my father and mother ultimately means that we give up impossible, self-destructive expectations. Until we learn to honor ourselves, we cannot truly honor our elderly parents."

Vivian felt compelled to ensure that her mother's every need was being taken care of. Until her mother pointed it out, she didn't realize that she was actually taking away what independence her mother had left. It's not uncommon for caregivers to become so involved in providing care that they take over and don't realize what persons in care can still do for themselves and the personal satisfaction for them that can result. A caregiver may be depriving the person of the only independence he or she is able to retain.

Vivian's commitment to the care of her parents led to an exclusion of care for herself. She became obsessed with serving the needs of her parents, which left no time to attend to her personal needs. Many caregivers fall into this pattern. It is vital that a caregiver realize that self-neglect and ignoring other family and personal obligations can be damaging to one's own health and other commitments.

Vivian spoke of her caregiver experience as learning and accepting the reality that all humans at some time will die. In many conversations I've had with persons of all ages, I've met some who will not talk about death as they approach the end of their life. In a circumstance when a parent's life is nearing the end, a new awareness of mortality and comfort with such conversations often comes.

1. Share a story when you have been in a caregiving situation where you have assumed more responsibility than necessary, resulting in depriving some measure of independence for the person in care. How have you become aware of the situation and how did you remedy it when appropriate?

2. Share a story about someone taking on a family caregiver commitment to the exclusion of the person's family, children, and self. Has this unhealthy attitude been modified? If so, what person or experience helped the caregiver or yourself understand the need for change?

3. Sharing stories about caregiving experiences and learning is a useful practice. Have you been in such a group, or have you organized or led one? How has the group worked for those involved? How long has the group been meeting? If the group no longer meets, did participants agree at the group's formation to meet for only a certain amount of time, or did group members decide they no longer need that support?

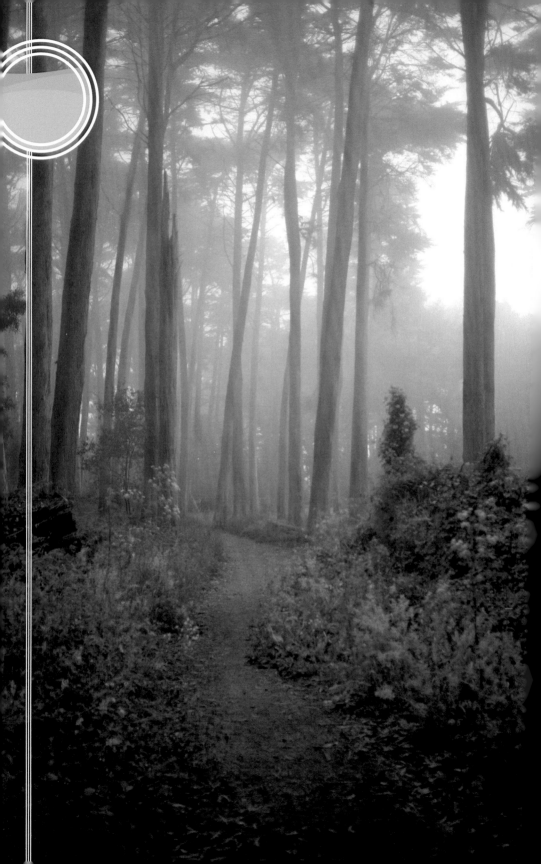

FAITH

WHAT I'VE LEARNED

ONE DAY MY PHONE RANG AND A FRIEND SAID, "I HEARD YOU'RE interviewing family caregivers. Here's my friend Faith's phone number. Call her." So I did, and she invited me to come over and talk. What might have seemed on the surface like an ordinary afternoon of tea and conversation was for me nothing ordinary at all. I was inspired by what Faith told me about her caregiver experience—what she learned and how she grew from it. I don't recall at what point in our conversation she repeated the words of Eleanor Roosevelt, but the quote captures the essence of Faith's caregiving story: "You gain strength, courage, and confidence by every experience in which you really stop to look fear in the face. . . . You must do the thing you think you cannot do." Shortly after she said that, I began recording her words.

We had always affectionately called my husband "Albert the absentminded professor," so I didn't think too much about his increasing lack of memory. Because he had always been a complete rebel, I rationalized that he just didn't care what others thought and didn't bother to remember what they said. Albert was a marvelous architect. He made the most beautiful designs. I was working then; my office was downtown in the federal building. I'd go to work and leave him at home to work on his drawings and plans.

Then strange things began happening. He flooded the kitchen with the garden hose. He began to wander and get lost. Albert was aware something wasn't right, and he was concerned about it. He became leery of strangers and was easily upset, even violent. The wandering became more frequent. Then he had a car accident. One day a friend was here visiting and quietly suggested to me, "Maybe you should take Albert for some neurological tests." The result was a diagnosis of Alzheimer's. I was devastated.

I tried to both work and manage Albert, but it wasn't long before I discovered that it was more than I could handle. To make a long story short, I quit my job to stay home and care for him. My son became concerned that I was exhausting myself and insisted I put Albert in a nursing home. Albert was in the home for about three months. It broke my heart to see him tied into a chair and on heavy tranquilizers; he was like a zombie. It was a hard choice for me to make, but I finally decided I would do everything I had to do to care for him at home. The day I picked him up and we pulled in front of the house, the first thing he said was, "I'm home, I'm really home."

It all seemed overwhelming. At first I had the thought, "What have I taken on? Can I do this?" Yet, in my heart I knew that for me it was the right thing to do. I tapered off his medications one at a time, and after a while I completely stopped all the drugs. I moved Albert into a room on the main level of the house and made it into a warm, welcoming area. I put posters on the wall and fresh flowers in the room, and there was a little deck outside where he could sit in the sun and have his meals. He gradually calmed down.

My husband couldn't feed himself very well, and soon he couldn't even talk. He lost the ability to walk and was falling all the time. He was a big, tall, strong man, so he needed help from someone who was also big and strong. Fortunately, I could afford to employ some male nursing assistants from a local agency to come in for a few hours each day, so I had some respite.

I began to realize that I had to have some time away, time to be refreshed, so I could come back and deal with it all. I began to go out to lunch, take a swim in the community pool, go shopping, or just take the dog for a walk. One thing I learned quickly was that to be a good and loving caregiver, you have to take care of yourself.

At some point rather early on I began keeping a diary. At the beginning, what was primarily on my mind was loss. The man I knew and loved and who had been a very important part of my life was gradually drifting away. The essence of this person I knew so well was eroding; he was quickly disappearing, and I needed to write about the loss. I also felt a need to write about the many wonderful things we had done together. I needed to focus on all those joyous and satisfying years we had shared. I'll never really lose him if I can hold on to what we had together. I'll always have these beautiful memories. I needed to write about my memories and feelings. My diary eventually became a book called *A Different Reality: An Alzheimer's Love Story.*

All forms of dementia are horrible, tragic. They rob a person of his or her personality; the whole essence of a person's being changes. The person you love disappears before your eyes. My comfort has come from my faith. It isn't the answer for everyone, but the Catholic Church gave me what I needed. I love the ritual and ceremony. It connects me to a Higher Power, and I personally need that. My faith gave me some peace and helped me through the whole experience.

Of course, my situation was a day-to-day struggle. Through it all I began to look at love in a different way, in a much deeper sense. So often when we think of love, the image that comes to mind is one of romance and joy. I began to wonder why we don't see beauty in some of those things about life that we usually perceive as ugly. For example, my husband's body was gradually coming apart; a beautiful, strong body was becoming old and feeble. Was this really something ugly? As I watched Albert fail and deteriorate, something touched my heart so deeply that I love him more than ever. I learned that the beauty of love is often in something that other people might call the ugly side of life, the side we don't want to see. To see that I loved Albert more completely, more honestly, more deeply than I ever thought possible was a dramatic transition for me. This change of perspective helped me get through the whole thing. I was so grateful that I could be there with him at this time of his life.

It was particularly hard as the end came near. A friend of mine suggested that I should contact our local hospice. Having their help was the most wonderful experience I have ever had. I can't say enough good things about hospice. They offered the understanding and sympathy we all needed. My family was here, friends came, and this small but close group surrounded Albert with love. Everyone was wonderfully supportive. I sat by him and held his hand, and he squeezed mine, opened his eyes, and said, "I love you." It was a peaceful death.

One of the most significant things I've learned from all this is that I'm strong. I never would have believed that before. I wasn't confident that I was competent, resilient, and strong.

Having gone through all this, having chosen the path of a caregiver, I'm much more secure and confident. I feel I can handle new challenges that may come into my life and find my new place in the world.

Many caregivers have told stories about a new understanding and deep growth between the family caregiver and person receiving the care, and many other lasting gifts such as confidence and personal strength. In Faith's situation, as her husband's dementia increased and his body weakened, her willingness to take on more of the caregiving responsibilities brought her unexpected confidence and a deeper love for her husband. Her caregiving also gave her new feelings of competence, resilience, and strength. I'm confident that Faith's story of newfound strength, courage, and personal growth is only one similar to millions told by others who have grown from their caregiver experience.

1. What was the message for you in Faith's story? How might you personally use or pass on to others what her story illustrates?

2. As Faith's husband's mind and body deteriorated, her love for him grew deeper. She also developed a deeper understanding of herself. When have you grown from a difficult experience? How did it change you?

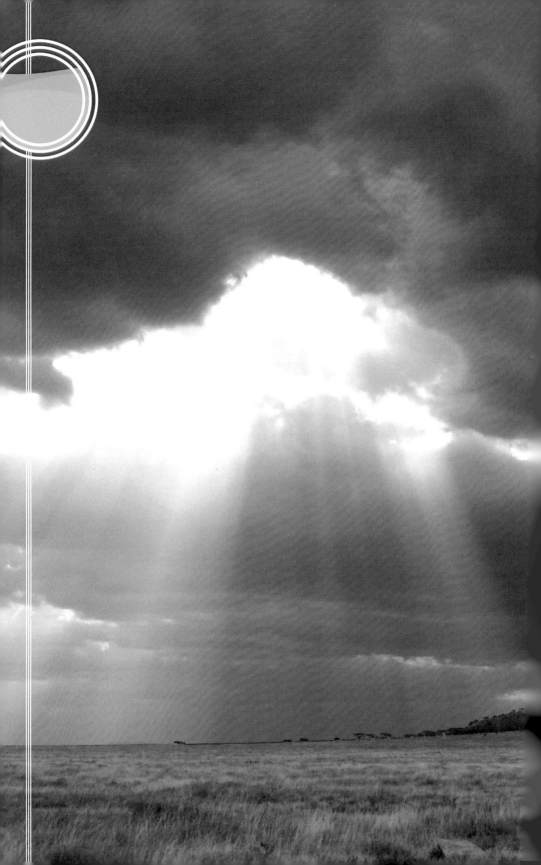

ALLEN

MY TEARS AND UNEXPECTED LAUGHTER

THE DEATH OF HIS YOUNG WIFE, ELLEN, PROFOUNDLY CHANGED Allen's life. Despite the fear, grief, and depression caused by Ellen's illness and suffering, Allen was led in the unexpected direction of laughter and humor. For several years now, Allen has called himself "the world's only jolly-ologist." In his speeches around the country and in the books he's written, he shows people how to use hope and humor to deal with the not-so-funny stuff: illness, caregiving, loss, depression, and grief. Allen and I talked together in the living room of his charming San Francisco home.

Ellen died here in our house. I brought her home from the hospital at around noon, and then went out to buy food. When I came back, Ellen's mother ran out of the bedroom with a pained look on her face and said, "I think Ellen has died." Ellen was on the floor. She had fallen out of bed. I put a pillow under her head and held her hand. Ellen's mother was frightened; she didn't know what to do. She asked whether should she call the undertaker. I said no. When our daughter came home from school, we all sat with

Ellen quietly for a while, and after some time had passed we called the funeral director. I know in these situations we all need some time. So we took the time needed to say good-bye to Ellen.

But that's the end of my caregiving story. Here's the beginning. We had just married and were living in New York City where I was freelancing as a scenic designer. We lived in an old tenement, and the landlord was trying to get us out. Only Ellen and I and one other tenant were left. One night a mysterious fire broke out. It was scary, but no one was hurt. The next morning the landlord gave us a big lump of money and said we should leave. I'd always wanted to live in San Francisco; it was my dream. I didn't have a job waiting, but we just packed and left New York.

We moved on a Thursday, and on Friday I went to the San Francisco Opera, told them I was a scenic designer, and asked if they needed help. They told me they were desperate for what I could offer, and I started working the following Monday. We found this wonderful Victorian house that we're sitting in now. I had always wanted to live in one and Ellen had too. I remember that I used to sit and draw pictures of Victorian houses when we were living in New York.

We had been in San Francisco about a year when Ellen went for a regular checkup, and the doctor said something was wrong. They did some blood tests, and it turned out to be a rare liver disease. There was no cure. At that time, 1975, only five liver transplants had been done. The doctor said Ellen would live three years and, indeed, that was exactly how long she survived.

Ellen was gregarious and fun and had tons of friends. She always wanted to party. The doctor said she should be in bed, and Ellen said, "No, I'm going out dancing." She said she wanted to enjoy life. I would be upset that she wasn't taking care of herself, but she was determined to have fun. Once Ellen went into the bathroom and yelled that she was going to flush all her medications down the toilet. She was yelling, "Go down. Get out of here!" and she was laughing. I failed to see the humor. I couldn't laugh.

Ellen was ill for three years. She had several operations; it was a very difficult time for us. I felt like there was nowhere to turn, no one to talk to. I went to see a therapist, and after the second session he told me, "Life is difficult." Neither my therapist nor her doctor gave us any hope. I desperately needed hope. Somehow, even though you know the person won't make it, hope gets you through day to day. As Ellen became more ill and her friends knew she was dying, I could count on one hand the number of people who came around to visit her. She was only thirty-one, and death frightened her peers, so a lot of them disappeared. Ellen was thin and yellow, and they didn't want to see her like that. Her friends only wanted to see the happy, outgoing Ellen.

When we were living in New York, a lot of our friends were separating and divorcing, and Ellen and I would ask each other, "Why are we still married?" Ellen would say, "You make me laugh." And that was one of the wonderful things about our relationship. We laughed a lot. It was a glue that held us together. But now I couldn't laugh.

Then one day while I was visiting Ellen in hospital, she handed me the centerfold from the latest *Playgirl* magazine and asked me to put it up on the wall. I said, "Ellen, I can't do that—this is a hospital." And she said, "Okay, then get a big leaf off the plant over there and cover up 'that part.'" So I did, and it was fine for the first and second days, but by the third day the leaf had shriveled up, and what we had tried to hide was showing. We both laughed. It was only five or ten seconds of laughter, but it helped me get another perspective.

This was the beginning of how a scenic designer became what I call a jolly-ologist. It gradually became clear to me that most people don't see the humor even when it is there. I now give talks and facilitate workshops at hospitals, nursing homes, churches, and other organizations on the value of humor in the midst of illness, suffering, and death. Most of the time when I give my talks, I come onstage with a red clown nose either on my face or in my pocket. The groups I address are quite different from one another. I try to judge at what point in my performance the nose gimmick would best work to relax and engage each specific audience. When the event is over, I stand by the door to talk with those who want to exchange comments or stories, and I give everyone a red clown nose of their own.

Once, my daughter encouraged a friend of hers, a rather depressed young man, to come to my talk. I spotted him reclining shyly at the rear of the room. As he left the room, he hastily grabbed a clown nose from my hand while I was engaged in conversation. Many months later my daughter told me he, feeling deserted and hopeless, had been contemplating suicide. He told her how late one night as he stood in front of the bathroom medicine chest, he reached into his pocket and pulled out that clown nose. Without thinking, he put it on his face and saw his reflection in the mirror. Seeing himself looking silly brought a spontaneous laugh. The deep gloom he had been feeling lifted just enough to cause him to change his plan. "Tell your father that his clown nose may have saved my life," he told my daughter. The stories I tell often lighten some very dark situations.

My father-in-law developed brain cancer and was hospitalized several times. For his and my mother-in-law's wedding anniversary, I suggested we have a small dinner party. I'd make a turkey and whatever else they wanted to serve and bring over. My father-in-law was enjoying the meal, but he was starting to doze off at the table. He didn't hear so well, so my mother-in-law passed him a note. She laughed as he read it, and he laughed too. She had written, "Happy Anniversary, dear. Do you want to go to bed?" He very lovingly and quietly leaned over and said to her, "I'd love to, dear, but we have company."

Death and dying are not funny, but funny things do go on even in the process of death and dying. When my dad passed away several years ago, my brother and I flew to Florida to sit shivah with my mom. As I walked into my parents' home, I heard Mom on the phone with the rabbi, telling him that her sons were there with her. But she got tongue-tied and said, "My other son is going back to Connecticut to shit siver." We all broke into laughter. We howled so much she couldn't talk and had to hand me the phone. I pulled myself together enough to tell the rabbi we'd call him back.

When I was taking care of Ellen, I often wished that a friend would come around to take me to a funny movie or play where I could laugh a little. Now I understand that caregivers need to find a bit of humor, some brief time out from the constant pressure and stress. Toward the end of Ellen's life I was running out of steam. Everything I did was for Ellen or my daughter. I didn't take very good care of myself. And I didn't understand that a good laugh could relieve stress or that a humorous perspective could lighten my burden. Many people have told me stories of laughter in the midst of loss, and I'm convinced that some Higher Power puts in some humor along with the hardship to help us through.

This understanding has had a profound influence on my life; it changed my career. I never imagined that I'd get up in front of an audience of people dealing with sickness and death and get them to laugh! I practically failed speech in college. But I realized I had a message about humor and loss, and every time I get up to speak, it's a personal healing. There's always humor all around us. When we're so busy being caregivers, we may not see it, but it is there; we only need to stop for a moment to embrace it. I realize when you're deeply involved in caregiving for a loved one, it's like you're wearing blinders. My challenge is to show people there is humor and hope.

The greatest lesson I learned from my caregiving experience was to be, just to be, with Ellen. So many people think they have to do something. You don't have to do anything but sit with your loved one. I learned from being with Ellen how to be with others. If sadness came up, we cried; if humor happened, we laughed.

I'm a better person for having been a caregiver. Those who have not yet experienced being around someone who is dying may not know that it makes you realize just how fragile life is. Every moment is precious. These valuable lessons are waiting to be learned, and you can smile, even laugh, while you're learning them.

I've often shared Allen's story when I've spoken at events for family caregivers and hospice providers. Many stay around after the event and tell me their experiences and stories of both hardship and humor.

I chose to place Allen's story at the end of this book for a specific reason. I know well the stresses, frustrations, sadness, and feelings of helplessness that are in every family caregiving situation. I've met and talked with so many who tell of circumstances that result in the death of the person in care. I've also collected stories of loved ones who have become permanently disabled and face a life of limitations. They share their moments of disappointment, despair, loss, and exhaustion, or of finding a new depth of unexpected awareness and profound learning. Yet they also share moments of unexpected laughter or of a simple smile that briefly eases the pain that is part of their lives.

1. Can you share a story when humor, at the right moment, brought balance into a depressing, possibly hopeless or prolonged situation? What specific realizations or change of mood and perspective was the result?

2. When has the use of humor been discussed in a training conference or seminar you have attended? What did you learn from this and how have you integrated humor into your work or personal life? If you have not discussed the use of humor, what is your opinion about the subject of appropriate humor being introduced in such trainings?

3. "I learned that laughter could walk into our lives when we least expect it." I don't know who said these words, but I've repeated that phrase many times. What stories or experiences can you share that validate the idea that humor can offer comfort at the appropriate time in a caregiving situation?

AFTERWORD
A CONVERSATION WITH STUDS TERKEL

AN AFTERWORD IS A BIT OF AN AUTHOR INDULGENCE. HOWEVER, because I feel so strongly about the power of story, I'm taking this opportunity to introduce Studs Terkel (1912–2008), one of the great American storytellers. This Chicago-based oral historian, radio personality, writer, and raconteur was as familiar to many of us as a favorite piece of comfortable furniture. You may have read his books or heard the nationally syndicated daily radio program he broadcast for many decades, or possibly you had an opportunity to meet him personally. Maybe you were among the many people he approached over the years with a request to share your hopes, dreams, fears, and feelings. "Tell me your story," Studs said hundreds of times as he turned on his tape recorder.

I met Studs Terkel in the late 1960s. I was just beginning what became for me a thirty-five-year career in educational and public radio. He was available for an interview at the University of Minnesota, where he was giving a lecture. I was a fledgling reporter at the campus radio station and was the lucky one assigned to interview him. Studs occasionally interviewed famous celebrities or well-known personalities, but he mostly collected stories of folks like you and me. Studs called these the stories of ordinary heroes. Yet, there's nothing ordinary or commonplace about the stories he collected. In the telling, these simply told, personal tales carry deep meaning, inspiration, and hope.

Studs Terkel's writings and his conversations with me are, for me, the ultimate proof of Muriel Rukeyser's observation, quoted in the introduction of this book: "The world isn't made of atoms, it's made of stories." The experiences of others have the power to affect us profoundly. But the mystical, magical power of stories is that they tell us not only about others but also about ourselves. People may be of a different race, religion, or economic status. They may be faced with a situation that has nothing to do directly with our lives. Yet the feeling, determination, acceptance, compassion, grit, and wisdom of their personal stories speak to us. Through these stories we gain insight, courage, comfort, and inspiration.

As I wrote the words above, I had just come back from a trip to Chicago where I had visited with Studs. He had invited me to come to his home. Of course, I brought along my tape recorder. "May I interview the interviewer?" I asked. "Sure, we can talk," he said. "But you know I generally don't talk about personal things." I was aware that Ida, his wife of sixty years, had died recently while undergoing heart surgery. On the window ledge in the living room was an urn holding her ashes. Next to it was a vase of yellow daisies, her favorite flower. He repeated to me what he had written in the introduction to his most recent book: "Sometimes I look over at the urn and mumble, 'Whaddya think of that, kid?'" Somewhat unwillingly, yet moved by his natural generosity, Studs began to talk about Ida.

She was eighty-seven when she died. We were married sixty years. For me Ida wasn't an old woman. She was that girl, that social worker in a maroon smock, that I first saw all those years ago, when I was doing some work for the WPA during the Great Depression. She would listen to clients tell their troubles. Ida was so open that people were just drawn to her. I learned that from her—a certain kind of awareness of others, a recognition of their feelings. She was like a dancer, light and delicate, yet strong. I remember what the poet Gwendolyn Brooks, who knew her well, said of Ida: "She could dance on a moonbeam." There was a wonderful grace about her. When she fell down, she'd say, "I fall gracefully." She bore pain gracefully. Even after her sense of taste was completely gone, we'd be at a dinner party and there would be an easiness about her. Like I say, there was a grace about her.

Ida had a heart valve operation and a bovine valve replacement many years ago. After fifteen years, it just wore out and there was a leakage. The doctors wanted to have surgery quickly. Thinking back I believe I talked her into the surgery. I remember the night before the operation she said, "I want to go home." She was really against having the surgery. I guess this is my confession that I should have listened to Ida and heard what she was saying. She was ready to go, yet she never, never complained. She knew she was dying. She wanted to go home. I don't think I'll say much more about Ida. I don't talk much about personal things.

Studs looked pensively at the urn on the window ledge. I recall a brief silence. We continued our conversation on another subject.

My last book, *Will the Circle Be Unbroken,* is about death, but it's really about life. A guy called me from Kansas City. He had read my book and was affected by one particular story about the illness and death of a loved one. He had lost his companion, and he told me that reading stories about other people dealing with sickness, suffering, and loss was a healing experience for him. Now he may go out and tell others his story and have an effect on someone else. People get insights this way.

I remember a story I included in an early book I did called *Working*. I had talked with this wonderful waitress, and she told me about her day working at this steak house—the varicose veins, the headaches, and the exhaustion at the end of the day. Why was a middle-aged woman a waitress? She needed the cash, her daughter was in trouble, her son was on drugs, her husband had left her. One day a man stopped me on the street. He said, "I read your book and I want to tell you how I feel about that story of the waitress. I'm never going to speak to a waitress like I've done before." He had never seen life from her point of view. I had touched him, and his behavior.

Here's something I learned from Ida. It's about truth. When you do a book, you choose people who have a certain insight, a way of saying things that other people feel but can't say. They tell the truth of their experiences and feelings. How do I find them? Sometimes it's accidental, sometimes people tell me about someone they know, and sometimes it's someone I know.

One time after I had done a radio broadcast about race relations, a woman called me. She was furious. In a very upset tone she told me, "You're so smug, so righteous about your liberal attitudes. You remind me of my mother." Now that interested me, so I asked for her mother's phone number. The conversation I ended up having with her mother turned out to be an excellent interview that I included in one of my books. She was wonderful. Then one time I got into a taxi, and the driver asked me if I had seen the movie *Lord Jim*. He was talking about the film based on Joseph Conrad's novel. And he said, "Well, that movie is about me. It's about a guy who was a coward all his life and suddenly found his courage. That's me."

I sensed it was a story too good to miss. I turned on my tape recorder. So, there you are. You never know.

Like I told you earlier, the book that just came out is about death, but it's really about life. James Joyce wrote in *Finnegans Wake,* "You really accept death when you recognize the permanence of life." What people do and say can have permanence. Maybe the stories of others I tell will have a continuing life. One guy who read my book called me up and talked about how deeply he had been affected by the story I told. Now he may have an effect on someone else. What we do here on this earth, what we say here—our stories—stay here when we're gone.

———————————————

Sometimes the answers we seek come from unexpected places. This morning I was going through a collection of notes and clippings I had planned to file weeks ago but never got around to. As I was sorting, I wasn't totally concentrating on what I was doing. My thoughts were on writing the conclusion to this afterword. I wanted to leave you, the reader, with a few words of inspiration, encouragement, and insight. Quite unexpectedly I found the very words I needed scribbled on one of the papers I was sorting. About five years ago I had read a book by Jean Shinoda Bolen entitled *Closer to the Bone.* She had written extensively and eloquently about life-threatening illness and the search for meaning. The book was impressive and I had taken many notes. Now, here on the back of an envelope, I found one of them. Bolen had quoted from a children's book by Barry Lopez called *Crow and Weasel* the following words. I leave you with Lopez's wisdom and insight:

> If stories come to you, care for them. And learn to give them away where they are needed. Sometimes a person needs a story more than food to stay alive.

ABOUT THE AUTHOR

Connie Goldman is an award-winning radio pro-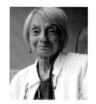
ducer and reporter. Beginning her broadcast
career with Minnesota Public Radio, she later
worked for several years on the staff of National
Public Radio in Washington D.C. For over the
past 30 years her public radio programs, books, and speaking
have been exclusively concerned with the changes and challenges of aging. Grounded in the art of personal stories collected
from hundreds of interviews, Connie's presentations are designed
to inform, empower, and inspire. Her message on public radio, in
print and in person is clear—make any time of life an opportunity
for new learning, exploring creative pursuits, self-discovery, spiritual deepening, and continued growth.